T0223010

Endovascular Tools & Techniques
Made Easy

Endovascular Tools & Techniques *Made Easy*

Edited by

Vikram S. Kashyap, MD, FACS

Professor, Surgery, Case Western Reserve University
Chief, Division of Vascular Surgery and Endovascular Therapy
Alan H. Markowitz MD Endowed Chair in Cardiovascular Surgery
Co-Director, Vascular Center,
Harrington Heart and Vascular Institute
University Hospitals Cleveland Medical Center
Cleveland, Ohio

Matthew Janko, MD

Resident Physician, Integrated Vascular Surgery
Division of Vascular Surgery and Endovascular Therapy
University Hospitals Cleveland Medical Center
Cleveland, Ohio

Justin A. Smith, MD

Resident Physician, Integrated Vascular Surgery
Division of Vascular Surgery and Endovascular Therapy,
University Hospitals Cleveland Medical Center
Cleveland, Ohio

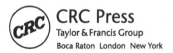

CRC Press
Taylor & Francis Group
Boca Raton London New York

CRC Press is an imprint of the
Taylor & Francis Group, an **informa** business

First edition published 2021
by CRC Press
6000 Broken Sound Parkway NW, Suite 300, Boca Raton, FL 33487-2742
and by CRC Press

2 Park Square, Milton Park, Abingdon, Oxon, OX14 4RN

© 2021 Taylor & Francis Group, LLC

CRC Press is an imprint of Taylor & Francis Group, LLC

Library of Congress Cataloging-in-Publication Data

Names: Kashyap, Vikram S., editor. | Janko, Matthew, editor. | Smith, Justin A., editor.
Title: Endovascular tools and techniques made easy / edited by Vikram S. Kashyap, Matthew Janko, Justin A. Smith.
Description: First edition. | Boca Raton : CRC Press, 2020. | Includes bibliographical references and index. | Summary: "This book complements and supplements the daily hands-on learning of residents and fellows in the areas of vascular surgery, interventional radiology, and interventional cardiology as they explore the world of endovascular and catheter-based procedures. Due to the complexity and growth in this field, it is vital that trainees establish a firm foundational knowledge of the basic construction of the tools they will be using, the properties that make them suited for addressing specific diseases, and their proper handling so that procedures can be completed effectively and safely"-- Provided by publisher.
Identifiers: LCCN 2020027794 (print) | LCCN 2020027795 (ebook) | ISBN 9780367279899 (hardback) | ISBN 9780367262426 (paperback) | ISBN 9780429299056 (ebook)
Subjects: MESH: Endovascular Procedures | Handbook
Classification: LCC RD598.5 (print) | LCC RD598.5 (ebook) | NLM WG 39 | DDC 617.4/13--dc23
LC record available at https://lccn.loc.gov/2020027794
LC ebook record available at https://lccn.loc.gov/2020027795

ISBN: 9780367279899 (hbk)
ISBN: 9780367262426 (pbk)
ISBN: 9780429299056 (ebk)

Typeset in Berling
by KnowledgeWorks Global Ltd.

To Sangeeta, Kate, and Kristy who have supported
and inspired us to achieve our goals.

Vik, Matt, and Justin

CONTENTS

CONTRIBUTORS

Ravi N. Ambani
Division of Vascular Surgery and Endovascular Therapy
University Hospitals Cleveland Medical Center
Cleveland, Ohio

Cassandra Beck
Department of Vascular Surgery
Cleveland Clinic Foundation
Cleveland, Ohio

Hiram Bezerra
Cardiovascular Imaging Core Laboratory
Interventional Cardiology Center
Harrington Heart and Vascular Institute
University Hospitals Cleveland Medical Center
Cleveland, Ohio

Saideep Bose
Division of Vascular Surgery and Endovascular Therapy
University Hospitals Cleveland Medical Center
Cleveland, Ohio

Teresa Carman
Division of Vascular Surgery and Endovascular Therapy
University Hospitals Cleveland Medical Center
Cleveland, Ohio

Jae S. Cho
Division of Vascular Surgery and Endovascular Therapy
University Hospitals Cleveland Medical Center
Cleveland, Ohio

Benjamin Colvard
Division of Vascular Surgery and Endovascular Therapy
University Hospitals Cleveland Medical Center
Cleveland, Ohio

Jon C. Davidson
Department of Interventional Radiology
University Hospitals Cleveland Medical Center
Cleveland, Ohio

David Hardy
Department of Vascular Surgery
Cleveland Clinic Foundation
Cleveland, Ohio

Karem C. Harth
Division of Vascular Surgery and Endovascular Therapy
University Hospitals Cleveland Medical Center
Cleveland, Ohio

Elder Iarossi Zago
Cardiovascular Imaging Core Laboratory
Harrington Heart and Vascular Institute
University Hospitals Cleveland Medical Center
Cleveland, Ohio

Matthew Janko
Division of Vascular Surgery and Endovascular Therapy
University Hospitals Cleveland Medical Center
Cleveland, Ohio

Vikram S. Kashyap
Case Western Reserve University
Division of Vascular Surgery and Endovascular Therapy
Harrington Heart and Vascular Institute
University Hospitals Cleveland Medical Center
Cleveland, Ohio

Ann Kim
Division of Vascular Surgery and Endovascular Therapy
University Hospitals Cleveland Medical Center
Cleveland, Ohio

Sami Kishawi
Department of Surgery
University Hospitals Cleveland Medical Center
Cleveland, Ohio

Norman H. Kumins
Division of Vascular Surgery and Endovascular Therapy
University Hospitals Cleveland Medical Center
Cleveland, Ohio

Jun Li
Department of Interventional Cardiology
Division of Cardiovascular Medicine
Harrington Heart and Vascular Institute
University Hospitals Cleveland Medical Center
and
Department of Medicine
Case Western Reserve University School of Medicine
Cleveland, Ohio

Eric McLoney
Division of Vascular and Interventional Radiology
Department of Radiology
University Hospitals Cleveland Medical Center
Cleveland, Ohio

Ryan Moore
Department of Surgery
University Hospitals Cleveland Medical Center
Cleveland, Ohio

Gabriel Tensol Rodriguez Pereira
Cardiovascular Imaging Core Laboratory
Harrington Heart and Vascular Institute
University Hospitals Cleveland Medical Center
Cleveland, Ohio

John "Will" Perry
Department of Vascular Surgery
Cleveland Clinic Foundation
Cleveland, Ohio

Mehdi Shishehbor
Department of Interventional Cardiology
Division of Cardiovascular Medicine
Harrington Heart and Vascular Institute
University Hospitals Cleveland Medical Center
Cleveland, Ohio

Justin A. Smith
Division of Vascular Surgery and Endovascular Therapy
University Hospitals Cleveland Medical Center
Cleveland, Ohio

Christopher Smolock
Department of Vascular Surgery
Cleveland Clinic Foundation
Cleveland, Ohio

Jason Ty Turner
Division of Vascular Surgery and Endovascular Therapy
University Hospitals Cleveland Medical Center
Cleveland, Ohio

Lisa Walker
Division of Vascular and Interventional Radiology
Department of Radiology
University Hospitals Cleveland Medical Center
Cleveland, Ohio

Virginia L. Wong
Division of Vascular Surgery and Endovascular Therapy
University Hospitals Cleveland Medical Center
Cleveland, Ohio

Ahmad Younes
Division of Cardiovascular Medicine
Harrington Heart and Vascular Institute
University Hospitals Cleveland Medical Center
and
Department of Medicine
Case Western Reserve University School of Medicine
Cleveland, Ohio

George K. Zhou
Case Western Reserve University School of Medicine
Cleveland, Ohio

PREFACE

We have witnessed an amazing evolution of treatment of patients with cardiovascular diseases with increasing utilization of minimally invasive endovascular therapies. The world of endovascular tools and techniques is vast, rapidly increasing, and can be confusing. In order to build a working knowledge of the myriad tools in this trade, one needs a firm foundation in understanding the purpose, technical parameters, and function of each tool. **Our goal in writing this handbook was to produce a practical resource on how to handle and use the tools, devices, and implants for endovascular interventions.** A multidisciplinary and diverse group of authors, including vascular surgeons, interventional cardiologists, and interventional radiologists, highlight their unique skills and expertise in this handbook.

We hope that this handbook helps individuals at all levels. Medical students, trainees, and physicians starting in practice will enhance their endovascular knowledge, which will allow for improved and seamless patient care. Even the experienced practitioner may find new tips in this book! Keep this text handy in the pocket of your white coat or scrubs (or on your phone!) and refer to it when questions come up about contrast dose, correct guidewire choice, basics of IVUS, and so on. We sincerely hope that this book helps you provide effective care for your patients with cardiovascular disease. We also hope it inspires you to spur further innovation in endovascular techniques that will help all of our patients.

CHAPTER 1

INTRODUCTION TO THE ENDOVASCULAR SUITE AND BASIC PRINCIPLES OF ANGIOGRAPHY

Jason Ty Turner, Virginia L. Wong

LEARNING OBJECTIVES

- Become familiar with typical equipment, personnel, devices, and workflow utilized in a Cardiac Catheterization Laboratory or a hybrid operating room
- Become familiar with nomenclature and basic concepts of fluoroscopy
- Understand the basic principles of angiography and radiation safety

Recently, there have been rapid advancements in endovascular technologies to treat arterial, venous, neurologic, and cardiac pathologies. These interventions commonly take place in an endovascular suite, such as a Cardiac Catheterization Lab (commonly referred to as the "Cath Lab") or a hybrid operating room equipped with fixed (permanently mounted) fluoroscopic imaging equipment. Other venues with similar equipment are "Interventional Radiology Special Procedures" area, and outpatient angiography areas (office-based lab/OBL, ambulatory surgery center/ASC, etc.). Interventions can be performed at body sites remote from the point of vascular access using fluoroscopy to guide the real-time passage of wires, catheters, and devices to those sites for treatment. **For simplicity, we will use endovascular suite as a generic term to encompass all venues where endovascular procedures, including angiography and intervention, can be performed.**

A number of team members work together in the endovascular suite, and each has a specific role and responsibilities:

- **Interventionalist (or Operator):** A physician specialist trained to perform endovascular procedures and responsible for the conduct of the case, safety processes, supervision of other team members, and management of complications. Often, the interventionalist directs patient sedation, while a separate individual, such as a circulating nurse or an anesthetist, monitors patient comfort and vital signs during the case.
- **Conscious Sedation Nurse:** A nurse specialist who may manage all aspects of patient sedation and monitoring. In some venues (such as hybrid operating room [OR]) an **anesthesiologist** may provide sedation, particularly for more complex cases.
- **Circulating Nurse:** This individual monitors the patient's condition, gathers supplies and opens equipment onto the sterile field, and performs point-of-care testing (e.g., blood glucose, activated clotting time) when needed.
- **Radiation Technologist:** A trained and licensed individual who operates fluoroscopy equipment and assists the interventionalist in handling wires, catheters, and devices during the case.
- **Recording Nurse or Tech:** This individual monitors the entire procedure from a separate control room, documenting the timing and conduct of each procedure step, the equipment used, and other important procedural parameters. A recording nurse or tech more often assists an interventionalist in a Cath Lab setting.

Generally, all team members assist with loading the patient onto the table and preparing to start the case, as well as with patient transfer to the recovery room afterward, and then room turnover for the following case. Good teamwork and clear communication are essential for maintaining a smooth workflow and safe environment for the patients and staff during the procedure.

Initial Procedural Workflow

Patients are typically prepared for their procedure in a pre-procedural area. Medical history, vital signs, and pertinent lab values are reviewed; consent for the procedure is obtained; and intravenous access secured. The patient is then brought to the endovascular suite (Figure 1.1) and placed on the procedure table. Hemodynamic and cardiorespiratory monitoring are established and supplemental oxygen is provided. Following institutional pre-procedural patient identification protocols, the appropriate body part is exposed, prepped into a sterile field, and intravenous sedation is administered.

Vascular access is most often achieved percutaneously with the modified Seldinger technique, using ultrasound or fluoroscopy to guide introduction of a needle into the vessel lumen. Surgical exposure of the access vessel via cut down approach can also be employed and is common during combined open and endovascular procedures performed in a hybrid OR. A guidewire is advanced through the access needle that serves as a rail, or pathway, for other devices such as sheaths and catheters to follow. These items can be advanced along the wire to various distant sites for intervention, using fluoroscopy to visualize their progress and position inside the body.

Procedural Imaging Step-by-Step

1. Typically, **fluoroscopy** is utilized for visualizing through body tissues and structures. Stepping on a foot pedal activates the imaging system. A single fluoroscopic image captured by simple press-and-release of the pedal is referred to as a spot image.

2. Blood vessels and the blood contained within them have the same radiodensity as other soft tissues, and so are not visualized with plain fluoroscopy. Therefore, radiodense **contrast dye** is administered into the vessel lumen to provide differentiation from surrounding tissues and allow them to be seen. There are a number of common contrast agents with varying characteristics, rendering each particularly useful for certain applications (see Chapter 4, "Contrast Agents and Their Delivery").

3. Contrast dye may be either **hand injected**, using a syringe attached to an intraluminal catheter, or **power injected**, using a specific mechanical injector. A **power injector** is capable of administering much greater volumes of contrast at a higher rate and pressure than is possible by hand, and so is useful when trying to fill a large vessel or one with rapid blood flow (such as the aorta) with contrast. The power injector must be programmed with the desired rate of contrast administration (milliliters per second) and the total amount of contrast volume (mL) to be injected. This conventional programming sequence results in the common expression for communicating power injector settings to other team members, where "10 for 20" means that a 20 mL volume of contrast will be injected at a rate of 10 mL per second. Other injection parameters such as pressure, rise, and delay can be set separately.

4. Prolonged pedal activation will capture and display multiple images using pulse dose fluoroscopy, with a frame (image capture) rate that is adjustable. A slower frame rate, such as 2–3 frames/second, is selected

when using fluoroscopy to aid navigation of wires, catheters, and other devices. Imaging rapid movements or changes in position requires a higher frame rate. **Cineangiography**, or a cine run, is a series of successive X-ray images typically obtained at 15–30 frames/second and is used to capture the movement of radiopaque contrast injected into vessels.

5. **Digital subtraction angiography** (DSA) uses an algorithm to digitally subtract out radiopaque structures from images obtained during a cine run. This is useful for obtaining isolated views of contrast-enhanced vessels without visual interference by adjacent or overlying bony structures and other radiodense materials such as orthopedic hardware, arterial calcification, metallic vascular stents, etc. The pre-contrast image, or mask, is obtained during the first few seconds of DSA exposure, then subtracted from subsequent frames of the same cine run. Contrast is then injected and appears radiodense on a background devoid of competing radiopaque structures. Road mapping is a technique used to overlay a DSA image of contrast-enhanced vessels on top of live pulse dose fluoroscopy, thus providing a live map for guidance of wires and devices in the vessel. Some advanced systems have the capability to pair live fluoroscopic imaging with pre-procedural computed tomography (CT) scans, further enhancing aided navigation in more complex procedures. The use of special fluoroscopy modes improves identification of vascular pathology and can help minimize the amount of radiation and contrast used during a procedure.

The fluoroscopy **procedure table** allows for movement of the patient in several axes (Figure 1.2). A mushroom-shaped knob on the tableside control panel is depressed to unlock and then "float" the tabletop over its support in the X and Y planes. A separate control raises or lowers the height of the tabletop in the Z plane, while tilted positions such as side-to-side "airplane" or "cradle" and Trendelenburg or reverse Trendelenburg can be achieved as well. Another set of controls moves the C-arm in various directions, independent of table position. The C-arm can spin in an arc over the patient from left to right, or it can tilt in a cranial-caudal axis to achieve oblique views of relevant anatomy. The C-arm may be positioned on either the left or right side of the table, across the horizontal (transverse) axis of the patient's body, or it can swing 90 degrees to the end of the procedure table over the patient's head and chest. Additionally, a ceiling-mounted C-arm can travel the length of the procedure table along its ceiling rails. Newer advanced C-arm systems are mounted on a flexible or jointed set of ceiling-mounted arms that allow for any angle of approach over the procedure table (Table 1.1).

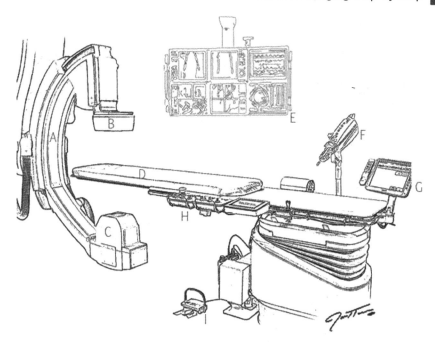

Figure 1.1 Key components of the endovascular suite. (A) C-arm. (B) Image intensifier (I-I). (C) X-ray source. (D) Procedure table. (E) Display screen. (F) Power injector. (G) Control panel for imaging system. (H) Tableside control for maneuvering table and C-arm.

Table 1.1 Endovascular Suite Design and Components

Component	Description
C-arm	Fluoroscopic imaging device, may be mounted on the ceiling or floor (Figure 1.1), comprised of an X-ray tube beneath the table and image intensifier ("I-I") above the patient
Procedure table	Radiolucent, can be moved independently in multiple planes
Display screen	Computer monitor or similar that shows live feed images and/or a static reference image received from the I-I, may also show physiologic data or imaging such as intravascular ultrasound (IVUS) or optical coherence tomography (OCT)
Back table (not shown)	Utilized for preparation of wires, catheters, sheaths, and other endovascular devices

5

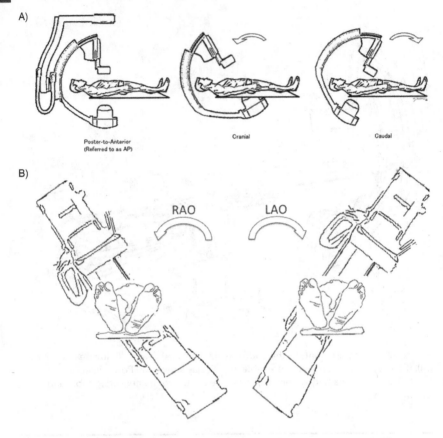

Figure 1.2 C-arm orientations. (A) Cranial-caudal orientations. (B) Oblique orientations.

The **standard angiographic imaging position** is with the C-arm placed in a perpendicular orientation over a supine patient, such that X-rays pass in a direct posterior to anterior (PA) direction. Technically, this is a radiographic PA view, although it is almost universally (and incorrectly) referred to as "AP," referring first to the location of the image intensifier (I-I) with respect to the patient, rather than that of the X-ray tube and direction of energy travel (see Figure 1.2). The nomenclature used for basic angiographic imaging positions refers to the angle of deviation from this direct AP position, again, using the I-I as the point of reference, with respect to the patient. Thus, if the C-arm is rotated to angle the I-I over the left side of the patient's body for a **left anterior oblique** (LAO) image, then the C-arm would be rotated to angle the I-I above the right side of the body for a **right anterior oblique** (RAO) image.

The degree of deviation from perpendicular can be specified for reference; for example, 30-degrees LAO means that the I-I has been rotated 30 degrees off of vertical toward the patient's left side. The C-arm can also be tilted in cranial or caudal directions, and these positions can be combined with right and left anterior oblique angles for viewing complex anatomy that cannot be distinguished in a standard AP plane of view (e.g., 20 degrees RAO and 10 degrees cranial-caudal).

Post-Procedure Workflow

After procedural completion, all devices are withdrawn from the patient using the appropriate closure technique. Techniques include manual compression of soft tissue over the puncture site (typically 5 minutes per sheath French size, followed by several hours of bed rest with the limb immobilized) or the utilization of a vascular closure device (see Chapter 14, "Post-Procedural Hemostasis and Closure Devices"). Open exposure of a vessel must be closed in standard surgical fashion. The most common complications after endovascular procedures involve the access point; including hematoma, arterial pseudoaneurysm, infection, dissection, and vessel thrombosis.

Being familiar with the components, personnel, and general terminology in the endovascular suite will help new team members assimilate easily into the workflow, no matter the institution or location of the endovascular suite within the facility (1, 2).

References

1. Killewich LA, Falls G, Mastracci TM, Brown KR. Factors affecting radiation injury. J Vasc Surg. 2011;53(1):9S–14S.
2. Stone PA, AbuRahma AF, Campbell JE. Vascular/Endovascular Surgery Combat Manual. 2012.

CHAPTER 2

PRE-PROCEDURAL RISK ASSESSMENT AND OPTIMIZATION

Sami Kishawi, Matthew Janko, Vikram S. Kashyap, Teresa Carman

KEYWORDS

risk assessment, patient optimization

LEARNING OBJECTIVES

- Recognize and assess patient comorbidities
- Understand risks associated with diagnostic or therapeutic catheter-based interventions
- Utilize various tools and strategies to assess a patient's peri-procedural risk of adverse event

Diagnostic and therapeutic catheter-based procedures have many benefits when compared with open surgery, including less physiologic stress, faster recovery, and less pain. However, these minimally invasive procedures still pose serious risks, such as exposure to contrast dye, unintended bleeding, and technical failure. It is essential to understand the risks of catheter-based procedures for each individual patient and to educate patients accordingly in a clear and understandable way. Furthermore, future interventions and unintended complications may require more invasive procedures, and thus it is essential to assess patients accurately at the time of their first (usually diagnostic) procedure.

Immediately Pre-Procedure

- Identify the patient's indication for the procedure.
- Obtain an accurate focused history of the patient's recent symptoms, including any recent illness, chest pain or pressure, or shortness of breath.
- Complete a focused physical exam with a thorough vascular exam to establish a baseline for post-procedure comparison. Importantly, all distal pulses or signals should be marked since catheterization of a more proximal vessel may result in thrombosis or embolism.
- Identify and review prior risk assessment and optimization documentation to confirm the patient is safe to undergo the planned procedure. This may include review of a recent note written by another medical professional stating the patient's risk, or perhaps noting the presence or absence of a diagnostic test. Particular attention should be paid to the patient's kidney function and to any allergy to contrast agent (see Chapter 4).

Cardiac Risk Assessment and Optimization

Peri-procedural adverse cardiac events include myocardial infarctions, arrhythmias, and perioperative heart failure. Today, the revised cardiac risk index (RCRI) is the most commonly used model for cardiac risk assessment in noncardiac surgery, especially in catheter-based procedures (1). Developed in 1999, this index identifies the following six risk factors:

- Ischemic heart disease
- Congestive heart failure
- Cerebrovascular disease
- Diabetes requiring insulin use
- Chronic kidney disease (creatinine >2 mg/dL)
- High-risk surgery

Risk for cardiac death or nonfatal cardiac event is based on the number of predictors present: 0 predictors, 0.4% risk; 1 predictor, 0.9% risk; 2 predictors, 6.6% risk; 3 or more predictors, >11% risk.

The following are the most common diagnostic studies used to assess heart structure and function.

1. **Electrocardiogram (ECG):** An ECG (often called EKG) is a non-invasive, inexpensive, and painless way to assess basic cardiac status. It is reasonable to establish a baseline ECG among any patient deemed to be at moderate to high risk. An ECG should be obtained to identify interval clinical changes if one is not available from the prior 6 months, or if any event has occurred since the most recent cardiac study. In the pre-procedural setting, ECGs are typically performed at rest and carry little value outside of providing additional context to a patient's baseline status (2). However, the ECG may be highly valuable post-procedure if there is a concern for cardiac event (3, 4).

2. **Echocardiogram:** An "echo" or "transthoracic echo" (TTE) is a non-invasive and painless way to assess heart function and pressures using ultrasound through the skin of the chest. The test can be augmented with medications or physiologic maneuvers, and can even be performed from within the esophagus (TEE). Echocardiography is appropriate to assess any moderate- to high-risk patients with the following:
   - A plan for complex or interventional procedures with the potential for blood loss or ischemia
   - A plan for diagnostic procedures to assess the function of the heart
   - A history of adverse cardiac event or recent cardiac intervention
   - A recent history of change of symptoms (i.e., new shortness of breath or angina) (3–5)

3. **Stress ECG or Echocardiogram:** A stress echocardiogram allows for evaluation of cardiac function and hemodynamic response to physiologic stress (6). Patients first undergo a baseline resting ECG, after which they undergo some form of stress. This is typically achieved through exercise (e.g., walking on a treadmill) or via intravenous medication (e.g., dobutamine), which acts to augment cardiac contractility and output mimicking exercise by increasing oxygen demand. Myocardial ischemia can be perceived by the patient as angina (chest pain), or visualized on ECG or on echocardiogram indicating the patient's inability to meet the hemodynamic demands of the procedure.

4. **Perfusion Scintigraphy:** In this test a radionuclide-labeled tracer, such as technetium-99m, is injected intravenously. Scintigraphy or single-photon emission CT captures images before and after cardiac stress. Changes in the distribution of blood flow to the heart can indicate compromised regional or focal myocardial perfusion. Presently, there is no clear superiority of one stress test or another in predicting cardiac risk; thus, utilization is based mostly on institution preference (7, 8).

Three types of medications – beta-blockers, aspirin, and statins – have demonstrated some degree of cardioprotection to decrease the peri-procedural risk of cardiac morbidity and ortality.

1. **Beta-Blockers:** β-adrenergic receptor antagonists including metoprolol, the most commonly used beta-blocker, act by blocking adrenergic receptors in the heart. This action decreases heart rate and contractility, and thus decreases oxygen demand and complications like ischemia, vasospasm, and inflammation (9). The 2014 American Heart Association recommendations state that patients on chronic beta-blocker therapy should continue taking beta-blockers through the peri-intervention period (6). Management of beta-blockers postoperatively, particularly in terms of dosing, should be guided by clinical circumstances. Patients with moderate to high cardiac risk may benefit from perioperative beta-blockers if they have not been started on any previously, but it is reasonable to initiate them days in advance to demonstrate safety and tolerability. Beta-blockers should not be initiated on the day of intervention because their safety and tolerability cannot be accurately assessed and because there is no evidence to suggest peri-procedural benefit (5–10).

2. **Aspirin:** Aspirin has antiplatelet, anti-inflammatory, and antipyretic properties through its inhibition of cyclooxygenase (COX). Among cardiac and vascular proceduralists and surgeons, it is commonly used with a second antiplatelet agent (e.g., Brilinta, Plavix, Effient) to reduce the risk of stent thrombosis. Typically, aspirin will be continued while the second agent is temporarily held (8). Low-dose aspirin use in the peri-procedural setting has been associated with decreased risk of myocardial infarction and should especially be continued in patients with coronary artery disease. Increased risk of bleeding is an adverse effect of aspirin, but this is generally considered to be low risk and not significantly contributory to major bleeding, especially in minimally invasive approaches.

3. **Statins:** Statins reduce cholesterol production, and thus the body's overall atherosclerotic burden and vascular inflammation. Long-term use has been shown to reduce major cardiac events, especially in patients with coronary artery disease. Similar to beta-blockers, withdrawal of statin use is associated with postoperative cardiac complication. Overall, statin use is widely favored as protective in the perioperative period.

Pulmonary Risk Assessment and Optimization

Chronic obstructive pulmonary disease (COPD, emphysema, asthma) and obstructive sleep apnea (OSA) are two of the most frequently encountered respiratory diseases in patients undergoing catheter-based interventions. Many patients have a smoking history or are active smokers. These patients are at risk of pulmonary complications and may benefit from pre-procedural assessment involving chest X-ray and OSA screening. The most common screening tool for OSA is the STOP-BANG questionnaire, and results may guide adjustments to anesthesia and hemodynamic monitoring [11]. These patients may benefit from pre-procedural medical therapy in the form of inhalers and/or continuous positive airway pressure therapy (CPAP).

Because opioid analgesics cause respiratory depression, judicious use of these medications in combination with multimodal alternatives is necessary to minimize post-procedural respiratory complications. Continuous pulse oximetry is a valuable procedural monitoring tool, and pre-procedural arterial blood gas analysis can assess for baseline hypoxia and/or hypercarbia.

Renal Risk Assessment and Optimization

Iodinated contrast media is commonly injected intravascularly during fluoroscopic procedures, yet is toxic to the kidneys and can cause contrast-induced nephropathy (CIN) in as many as 2% of patients with normal baseline kidney function. This risk increases in patients with pre-existing kidney disease [12]. In addition, renal perfusion may be altered by changes in hemodynamics, atherosclerotic embolization, or dissection causing an acute kidney injury. Besides intraoperative strategies to use dye conservatively, patients with reduced renal function should be given intravenous fluids prior to the administration of contrast dye and assessed for alternatives to iodinated contrast including carbon dioxide and coaxial intravascular imaging modalities if possible.

Hematologic Risk Assessment and Optimization

The most frequently encountered hematologic abnormalities among patients undergoing catheter-based procedures are anemia and thrombocytopenia. Patients are often on anticoagulant and/or antiplatelet therapies for various comorbidities, including prior deep vein thrombosis, atrial fibrillation, or prior intravascular stent. A pre-procedural complete blood count (CBC), basic chemistry panel, and coagulation panel including prothrombin time (PT)

Table 2.1 Common Antiplatelet and Anticoagulant Medications with Corresponding Reversal Agents

Agent	Mechanism of Action	Half-Life	Reversal Agent	When to Hold
Aspirin	COX inhibitor	6 hours	None	7–10 days
Clopidogrel	GPIIb/IIIa-complex inhibitor	6 hours	None	5–7 days
Warfarin	Inhibits Factors II, VII, IX, X, and protein C and S	25–60 hours	FFP, vitamin K, coagulation factors	Until INR normalizes
Enoxaparin	Anti-factor Xa and anti-IIa	4–6 hours	Protamine sulfate	12 hours
Apixaban	Direct factor Xa inhibitor	8–15 hours	Charcoal (if within 5 hours); Andexxa	5–7 days (if high risk of bleeding)
Rivaroxaban	Direct factor Xa inhibitor	10 hours	Charcoal (if within 2 hours); Andexxa	5–7 days (if high risk of bleeding)
Dabigatran	Direct thrombin inhibitor	10–15 hours	Charcoal (if within 2 hours); Praxbind	5–7 days (if high risk of bleeding)

Abbreviations: COX, cyclooxygenase; GP, glycoprotein; FFP, fresh frozen plasma; INR, International Normalized Ratio; II, two; VII, seven; IX, nine; X, ten.

and International Normalized Ratio (INR) are indicated for almost all patients pre-procedurally (8).

Antiplatelet or anticoagulant agents are sometimes held temporarily for elective cases. For more emergent cases, reversal agents may be necessary to normalize clotting times or restore clotting factors. Table 2.1 lists common agents and their appropriate reversal agents.

Summary

Outside of the inherent risks associated with any procedure, outcomes can be significantly altered by coexisting comorbid conditions that are not appropriately identified and optimized in the pre-procedural setting. Patients warrant risk stratification and optimization to predict and prepare for intra- and post-procedural adverse events. This is especially important since many patients that undergo endovascular procedures are deemed to be too high risk for surgical interventions. For these reasons, patients with significant comorbidities are often selected for minimally invasive endovascular interventions

---

Key Points

- Risk assessment begins with a focused history, physical exam, and review of systems.
- Emergent procedures should not be delayed by pre-procedural risk stratification and optimization.
- Cardiac risk assessment and optimization begins with an RCRI score and can involve ECG, echocardiography, and pharmacologic adjuncts (beta-blockers, aspirin, statins).
- Patients with COPD, OSA, and patients who smoke are at high risk of pulmonary complications.
- Consider pre-procedural hydration in patients with poor renal function or those at risk of contrast-induced nephropathy.
- Anticoagulant medications are frequently held prior to elective cases, whereas reversal agents may be necessary in emergency or unplanned cases.

References

1. Lee TH, Marcantonio ER, Mangione CM, et al. Derivation and prospective validation of a simple index for prediction of cardiac risk of major noncardiac surgery. Circulation. 1999;100(10):1043–9.
2. Poldermans D, Hoeks SE, Feringa HH. Pre-operative risk assessment and risk reduction before surgery. J Am Coll Cardiol. 2008;51(20):1913–24.
3. Goldman L, Caldera DL, Nussbaum SR, et al. Multifactorial index of cardiac risk in noncardiac surgical procedures. N Engl J Med. 1977;297(16):845–50.
4. Detsky AS, Abrams HB, Forbath N, Scott JG, Hilliard JR. Cardiac assessment for patients undergoing noncardiac surgery. A multifactorial clinical risk index. Arch Intern Med. 1986;146(11):2131–4.
5. Fleisher LA, Fleischmann KE, Auerbach AD, et al. ACC/AHA guideline on perioperative cardiovascular evaluation and management of patients undergoing noncardiac surgery: a report of the American College of Cardiology/American Heart Association Task Force on practice guidelines. J Am Coll Cardiol. 2014;64(22):e77–137.
6. Zarinsefat A, Henke P. Update in preoperative risk assessment in vascular surgery patients. J Vasc Surg. 2015;62(2):499–509.
7. Poldermans D, Schouten O, Bax J, Winkel TA. Reducing cardiac risk in non-cardiac surgery: evidence from the DECREASE studies. Eur Heart J. 2009;11(A Suppl):A9–14.
8. Sams S, Grichnik K, Soto R. Preoperative evaluation of the vascular surgery patient. Anesthesiol Clin. 2014;32(3):599–614.

9. Yang H, Raymer K, Butler R, Parlow J, Roberts R. The effects of perioperative beta-blockade: results of the Metoprolol after Vascular Surgery (MaVS) study, a randomized controlled trial. Am Heart J. 2006;152(5):983–90.

10. Devereaux PJ, Yang H, Yusuf S, et al. Effects of extended-release metoprolol succinate in patients undergoing non-cardiac surgery (POISE trial): a randomised controlled trial. Lancet. 2008;371(9627):1839–47.

11. Chung F, Subramanyam R, Liao P, Sasaki E, Shapiro C, Sun Y. High STOP-Bang score indicates a high probability of obstructive sleep apnoea. Br J Anaesth. 2012;108(5):768–75.

12. Zhan HT, Purcell ST, Bush RL. Preoperative optimization of the vascular surgery patient. Vasc Health Risk Manag. 2015;11:379–85.

CHAPTER 3

RADIATION SAFETY FOR YOU AND YOUR PATIENT

George K. Zhou, Justin A. Smith, Benjamin Colvard

KEYWORDS

radiation, scatter, fluoroscopy, shielding, ALARA

LEARNING OBJECTIVES

- Understand sources of radiation and the types of radiation used by interventionalists
- Understand the risks associated with radiation use and the necessity to minimize exposure to patient and care providers
- Be able to follow as low as reasonably achievable (ALARA) guidelines to reduce radiation exposure by minimizing time of exposure, maximizing distance from radiation sources, and with proper barrier utilization

Radiation is unavoidable in daily life as we all receive some level of background radiation from natural sources (e.g., ultraviolet light from the sun, radon gas, etc.). As an interventionalist, radiation is necessary for fluoroscopic imaging, as it allows for the diagnosis and treatment of patients, but it puts care providers at an increased risk for its adverse effects. Because of this, a fundamental understanding of this radiation, its effects, and how to protect radiation injury are vital to the health of caregivers and patients alike.

Types of Radiation

Radiation is energy that is emitted in the form of electromagnetic waves or particles. The types of radiation, and the energy that they possess, are often described in terms of their wavelengths, with shorter wavelength varieties having higher frequencies, and thus more energy. Categorically, radiation can also be split into **nonionizing versus ionizing radiation**, depending on whether those waves have enough energy to remove electrons from their targets (Figure 3.1).

Nonionizing radiation has longer wavelengths (>124 nm), lower frequencies (<3 × 10¹⁵ Hz), and thus lower energies, which are not sufficient to remove electrons from molecules or atoms (e.g., low-ultraviolet, visible light, infrared, microwaves, radio waves).

Ionizing radiation has shorter wavelengths (<124 nm), higher frequencies (>3 × 10¹⁵ Hz), and thus energy levels sufficient to interact with tissues by removing electrons from molecules or atoms (e.g., high-ultraviolet, X-rays, gamma rays). This is the radiation that is relevant to the interventionalist as X-ray is the means by which vessels and endovascular tools are imaged, which come with the risk of adverse biological effects with sufficient exposure.

Risks of Radiation

The biological effect and potential damage caused by ionizing radiation depends on the amount of energy absorbed and the sensitivity of the particular organ exposed. **Absorbed dose** refers to the quantity of energy from radiation absorbed per unit mass (Joules per kilogram); the unit for absorbed dose is the gray (Gy). Although absorbed dose can help us quantify radiation exposure, it does not reflect the extent of tissue damage because different tissues are

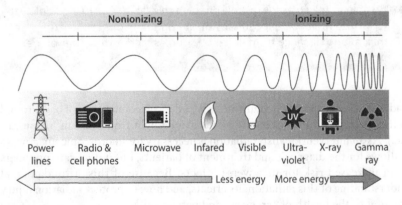

Figure 3.1 Spectrum of wavelengths of nonionizing and ionizing radiation.

differentially sensitive to damage by radiation. To quantify this, the term **equivalent dose** is used, which refers to the amount of biological damage incurred by a tissue/organ; the unit for equivalent dose is the sievert (Sv) and is directly proportional to the damage a tissue sustains from radiation. In most cases, gray and sievert are equivalent, with gray used to quantify radiation use for most endovascular procedures.

Ionizing radiation has the potential to damage cells, after which the cells will either successfully repair themselves, die, or acquire a mutation. Cellular damage following radiation can be classified into **deterministic and stochastic effects**.

Deterministic effects are dose dependent, with the chance that such an effect will arise, as well as the severity of that effect, being dependent on how much radiation is absorbed. Many deterministic effects generally require a minimum threshold of radiation absorbed to occur. This threshold varies among both tissues and individuals. Examples of deterministic effects include hair loss, skin necrosis, cataracts, congenital abnormalities (for radiation on pregnant mothers), and sterility (Table 3.1).

Stochastic effects are all-or-none; the probability of stochastic effects occurring is proportional to the dose absorbed, but once they occur, severity is generally not a function of radiation dosage. Unlike deterministic effects, these effects do not have a threshold. The main concern of stochastic effects is cancer. Many types of cancer are associated with radiation exposure, including leukemia, lungs, thyroid, breast, skin, gastrointestinal tract, and so forth. The probability of fatal cancer increases by 4% per Sv of lifetime dose.

Radiation in the Operating Room/ Angiographic Suite

X-rays in the operating room or angiographic suite are emitted via portable or floor-mounted C-arm machines. In these machines, X-ray photons are generated from an anode via its bombardment by electrons emitted from

Table 3.1 Deterministic Effects and Threshold Examples

Effect	Absorbed Radiation Dose (Gy)
Skin erythema	2–5
Irreversible skin damage/necrosis	20–40
Hair loss	2–5
Sterility	2–3
Cataracts	0.5
Lethality (whole body)	3–5
Congenital defects	0.1–0.5

an adjacent cathode (Figure 3.2A). The X-ray beam travels from the X-ray tube, through a focusing apparatus (collimator), through the patient, then to a digital detector (or image intensifier [I-I] in older devices), and finally hits the digital analyzer that generates an image (Figure 3.2B).

Despite the X-ray beam being the primary source of radiation exposure for the patient, it is not the case for the interventionalists and staff because they are usually standing away from the beam's direct path. **Scatter radiation** is the primary source of radiation exposure to care providers.

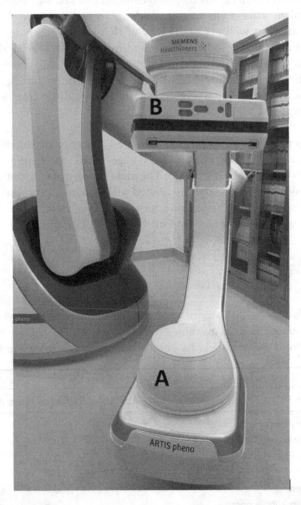

Figure 3.2 Example of floor-mounted, robotic arm-based C-arm X-ray. (A) X-ray source. (B) Image-intensifier/detector.

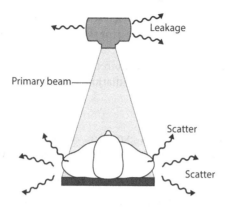

Figure 3.3 Sources of radiation exposure for patient and provider. Primary beam radiation, from the X-ray source directed at the patient, and leakage radiation, through the X-ray source housing, contribute to minor degrees. Scatter radiation, emanating from the patient, composes the primary source of exposure for the provider and is what shielding and radiation practices aim to protect against.

Scatter radiation When a radiation beam interacts with any substance, smaller amounts of radiation from that beam can bounce off in various directions. In the context of the operating room, the patient then becomes a secondary source of radiation via radiation scattered off their body from the primary X-ray source. Scatter radiation coming from the patient can affect nearby structures in the patient's body as well as increase radiation exposure to the operator (Figure 3.3).

Tools and Techniques to Protect from Radiation

Dose and Emission Control

Radiation dose can be directly decreased by managing the X-ray hardware. **Decreased current** and **increased voltage** of the X-ray tube can decrease radiation dose and usually does not affect image quality. Because X-rays are generated by a stream of electrons from a cathode bombarding an anode, decreasing the current (flow of electrons) from the cathode will decrease the dose of X-rays generated. Increasing voltage increases penetration of the beam and enhances contrast, which compensates for the decreased image resolution.

Larger image intensifiers can help generate the same image quality using less radiation. A **collimator** should also be used to focus the beam, which would both decrease leakage radiation and enhance image resolution. Collimators are composed of lead (or some other radiopaque material) shutters that can be adjusted to frame the region of interest to image and direct photons only to the area of interest; this focused beam then reduces radiation exposure to surrounding tissues.

Radiation safety practices are centered around the ALARA guidelines, which describe how to minimize radiation exposure using **time**, **distance**, and **barriers**.

For patients:

1. **Time:** Minimize the time of exposure. Avoid continuous activation of beam; instead, use short intermittent bursts of exposure. Note total fluoroscopy time and use it to calculate the patient's absorbed dose to ensure it does not exceed recommended values.

2. **Distance:** Place the patient as far from the X-ray tube and as close to the I-I as possible. Increasing distance between the patient and the X-ray tube decreases skin radiation. Placing the I-I closer to the patient allows us to maximize the quality of the image, thus requiring a lower dose. Raise the table and lower the flat panel detector (or I-I) close to the patient.

   Exposure is inversely proportional to distance from the X-ray source to the second power (exposure = $1/d^2$), meaning that doubling the distance will decrease exposure by a factor of 4.

3. **Barriers:** Barriers (lead or equivalent) should cover areas of the patient's body that are outside of the area of interest. For example, lead aprons can be worn by the patient for X-rays of the extremities.

For operator(s):

4. **Time:** Just like for the patient, minimize the time of exposure using ad hoc bursts instead of continuous activation.

5. **Distance:** Maximize the distance between the operator and both the X-ray tube (for leakage radiation) and patient (for scatter radiation). Many imaging apparatuses come with a control pad, or pedal system, either wireless or attached to a long cord to allow operators to stand far away from the source and patient and still operate the equipment during image acquisition. This is important during angiographic imaging of large vessels, or digital subtraction angiography (DSA) acquisitions, where the largest levels of radiation and longest exposures are used.

6. **Barriers:** These include table aprons and mobile shields.
   - **Table aprons:** Tableside lead shields positioned between operator and radiation source located beneath the table.
   - **Mobile shields:** Wheeled or ceiling-mounted shields that can be placed around the patient to reduce scatter to care providers in the room. These can be made with heavy metals (usually lead)

or leaded acrylic (transparent). Ceiling-mounted acrylic shields allow visibility and shielding together, and can reduce doses to the operator's brain and eyes by 20-fold.

Personal Protective Equipment

- **Aprons:** Traditionally made of lead, but they may include other heavy metals mixed in (e.g., barium, aluminum, tin, antimony, bismuth, tungsten, titanium) (6). The effectiveness of a shield is measured as "lead equivalent" and should be provided for each barrier.

  Lead garments usually range from 0.25- to 1.0-mm lead equivalent; 0.25 mm is the minimum recommended thickness, attenuating 96% of radiation dosage, whereas 0.5 mm attenuates up to 99%. Operators should always make sure the front of the apron is pointed at the radiation source when it is active. If it is essential to the procedure for the operator's back to face the radiation source, a wraparound garment should be used.
- **Thyroid Collars:** The thyroid is highly radiation sensitive, and frequent radiation to the thyroid increases the risk of thyroid cancer. Thyroid collars may limit movement due to their weight and size, compelling some interventionalists to omit them or wear them loosely. However, they are very effective at shielding the thyroid and should be diligently and properly worn; 0.5-mm lead equivalent thickness is recommended for thyroid collars (7).
- **Lead Glasses:** The lens of the eye is the most radiation-sensitive tissue of the body, and frequent radiation can lead to cataracts. Lead glasses should be used as an adjunct to mobile barriers as the eyes are still exposed to radiation from the sides of the head as the operator turns (1, 2). Most glasses contain 0.75-mm lead equivalent thickness.
- **Lead Caps:** Used as an adjunct to mobile shields and lead glasses, they can help protect the eyes and brain from radiation and further reduce risk of cataracts and brain cancer (1–4).
- **Protective Gloves:** Sterile protective surgical gloves can only provide 15–30% radiation attenuation. Protective gloves should be used if hands would be placed in the primary X-ray beam. However, operators should only put their hands in the X-ray beam when it is essential to the procedure.
- **Disposable Radiation Shields:** Sterile disposable pads can be placed over the patient to reduce scatter radiation. They can lead to 20% or more reduction in operator exposure (5).

  Finally, most states mandate that hospitals monitor radiation exposure using **dosimeters** to measure absolute dose received over time for operators. One should be worn at waist level under the lead apron, and another, external to the lead, on the thyroid shield.

Key Points

- Ionizing radiation in the form of X-rays is the type of radiation utilized in endovascular interventions.
  - Despite its benefits in diagnostic imaging and interventions, ionizing radiation can result in tissue damage and therefore unnecessary exposure should be minimized.
- The primary source of radiation exposure concerning interventionalists is scatter radiation emanating from patients as X-rays bounce off them from the X-ray source.
- Radiation exposure for interventionalists and patients is best minimized through adherence to the ALARA principles, which emphasize:
  - Time – Reducing the amount of time during imaging and interventions during which the radiation source is active.
  - Distance – Maximizing distance from the radiation source when it is active.
  - Shielding – Donning of appropriate lead garments and proper positioning of mobile shields to protect from scatter radiation when radiation sources are active.

References

1. Badawy MK, Deb P, Chan R, Farouque O. A review of radiation protection solutions for the staff in the cardiac catheterisation laboratory. Heart Lung Circ. 2016;25(10):961–967.
2. Schueler BA. Operator shielding: how and why. Tech Vasc Interv Radiol. 2010;13(3):167–171.
3. Kuon E, Birkel J, Schmitt M, Dahm JB. Radiation exposure benefit of a lead cap in invasive cardiology. Heart. 2003;89(10):1205–1210.
4. McCaffrey JP, Tessier F, Shen H. Radiation shielding materials and radiation scatter effects for interventional radiology (IR) physicians. Med Phys. 2012;39(7Part1):4537–4546.
5. Vlastra W, Delewi R, Sjauw KD, Beijk MA, Claessen BE, Streekstra GJ, Bekker RJ, van Hattum JC, Wykrzykowska JJ, Vis MM, Koch KT. Efficacy of the RADPAD Protection Drape in reducing operators' radiation exposure in the catheterization laboratory: a sham-controlled randomized trial. Circ Cardiovasc Interv. 2017;10(11):e006058.
6. Bates MC, Nanjundappa A. Radiation Safety. In: Stone PA, AbuRahma AF, Campbell JE, editors. Vascular Surgery Combat Manual. Flagstaff: W.L. Gore & Associates, Inc.; c2013. Chapter 5.
7. Cheon BK, Kim CL, Kim KR, Kang MH, Lim JA, Woo NS, Rhee KY, Kim HK, Kim JH. Radiation safety: a focus on lead aprons and thyroid shields in interventional pain management. Korean J Pain. 2018;31(4):244.

CHAPTER 4

CONTRAST AGENTS AND THEIR DELIVERY

Justin A. Smith, Jon C. Davidson

KEYWORDS

angiography, contrast agents, fluoroscopy

LEARNING OBJECTIVES

- Understand how contrast agents allow for angiographic imaging
- Understand how iodinated contrast agents function in allowing visualization of the blood vessel lumen and flow
- Know the indications, contraindications, and complications of contrast agents
- Understand the methods of contrast administration
- Appreciate an alternative to iodinated contrast, such as CO_2

Human tissues absorb X-ray photons to varying degrees (attenuation), and anatomy can be visualized by detecting those unabsorbed photons that have made their way through the tissue to a detector on the other side. However, differentiating neighboring tissue types requires that they possess sufficiently different degrees of attenuation. Without the aid of contrast agents, all elements of the vasculature demonstrate such similar attenuation to where differentiation of these structures is not possible on plain radiogram.

Contrast agents enable angiographic imaging due to their vastly different absorptive properties compared with body tissues. Iodinated contrast agents mix with flowing blood to fill the vasculature with material of vastly different X-ray absorption to allow us to accurately visualize the blood vessel lumen and blood flow patterns as we follow their path.

Contrast agents serve as powerful tools for imaging but should be thought of as a drug like any other with potentially deadly unintended effects.

Contrast Agents

Iodinated Agents: These are standard and commonly used. These agents are the go-to for their ability to mix with flowing blood and convey a high degree of X-ray attenuation (positive contrast), revealing a patient's vascular anatomy with superior image quality and accuracy over other contrast agents (e.g., CO_2) (1, 2). Despite the various manufacturers, brands, and formulations, all iodinated contrast agents are similar at the molecular level, composed of different variations of iodinated benzene. Such agents can be generally grouped into two broad categories, ionic and nonionic, based on whether they dissociate into anions and cations in solution with human blood. Clinically, this may be relevant for patients who may be sensitive to administration of hypertonic solutions (e.g., hypernatremia, intracranial processes) as many ionic contrast agents exhibit osmolality significantly higher (upward of 7–8×) than human plasma. Of additional clinical importance is the fact that administration of these agents effectively represents a dosage of iodine conveyed to patients during imaging, which can induce hyperthyroidism in patients who are iodine deficient or suffer from multinodular goiter. The concentration of iodine is often easily discernable for nonionic contrast agents from their names (e.g., Isovue®-200, Oxilan®-300, Ultravist®-370 contain 200, 300, and 370 mg/mL of iodine, respectively).

Contraindications

- History of prior allergic-type reaction to iodinated contrast. (**You must clarify the nature of any documented reaction for your patient!**) While the estimated prevalence of adverse reactions to iodinated contrast is 1–12%, severe, anaphylactic reactions make up only 0.01–0.2% of these (3)! For high-risk patients with these severe reactions, premedication regimens with corticosteroids and antihistamines are commonplace and can be administered within 12–13 hours prior to imaging (Table 4.1) (4, 5). In emergent circumstances, when premedication cannot be given and iodinated contrast agents are needed, patients should be closely monitored and anesthesia staff on hand to manage airway compromise.
- Severe, chronic renal impairment (estimated glomerular filtration rate [eGFR] < 30 mL/min/$1.73m^2$) without anuria and not on hemodialysis (while this is an absolute contraindication, **any degree of baseline renal dysfunction should be thought of as at least a relative contraindication and taken into consideration before a procedure**). Intravascular volume expansion with isotonic crystalloid (often 0.9% NaCl) is common practice for prevention of contrast-induced nephropathy

Table 4.1 Premedication Regimens for Patients with Prior Severe Allergic-Like Reactions to Iodinated Contrast

Hours Prior to Contrast Administration	Medications and Recommended Dosing	
	Regimen 1	*Regimen 2*
13	Prednisone 50 mg PO	
12		Methylprednisolone 32 mg PO
7	Prednisone 50 mg PO	
2		Methylprednisolone 32 mg PO
1	Prednisone 50 mg PO Diphenhydramine 50 mg OR 1 mg/kg PO/IM/IV	Diphenhydramine 50 mg OR 1 mg/kg PO/IM/IV

Abbreviations: IM, intramuscular; *IV,* intravenous; *PO,* by mouth.

Sources: Adapted from Sanchez-Borges M, et al. Controversies in Drug Allergy: Radiographic Contrast Media. J Allergy Clin Immunol Pract 2019. 7(1):61-65; and Beckett KR, Moriarity AK, Langer JM. Safe Use of Contrast Media: What the radiologist needs to know. Radiographics 2015. 35(6):1738-50.

in at-risk patients despite the absence of well-designed randomized clinical trials and with conflicting evidence in the current literature (Table 4.2) (6). Other prevention measures, including hydration with sodium bicarbonate solution and pre-procedure administration of N-acetylcysteine are practiced at some centers, although current literature has not demonstrated a benefit with these practices (7).

- Acute kidney injury.
- Thyroid disease (untreated Graves disease, multinodular goiter, suspected iodine deficiency before supplementation) (5).
- Close proximity to planned radioactive iodine therapy (contrast administration may interfere with efficacy of this therapy) (5).

Adverse Effects

- Allergic reaction
  - Contrast-induced nephropathy
- Hyperthyroidism (in patients with above-mentioned thyroid disease)

Contrast Injection

Manual Injection (Hand Injection): This simple method of contrast injection can be used to optimally image many medium and small blood vessels, where small amounts of contrast (<10 mL) are required. Injection can be performed with a

Table 4.2 Intravenous Hydration for Patients Undergoing Catheter-Based Angiography ± Intervention

Pre-Procedure	Intra-Procedure	Post-Procedure
CKD 3a (GFR 45–59): Have patient drink 6–8 glasses of water (8 oz) over 12–24 hours prior to procedure	1.0–1.5 mL/kg/hr 0.9% NaCl IV	1 mL/kg/hr 0.9% NaCl 6–12 hours
CKD 3b (GFR 30–44): 500 mL 0.9% NaCl over 4 hours prior to procedure. May need to be admitted prior to procedure		OR 6 mL/kg/hr 0.9% NaCl 4–6 hours
CKD 4+ (GFR < 30): RE-CHECK IMMEDIATELY. If accurate, report results to attending physician. Procedure may need to be canceled if the patient is not already on dialysis		

Abbreviations: CKD, chronic kidney disease; GFR, glomerular filtration rate; IV, intravenous.

simple Luer lock syringe containing full-strength or diluted contrast connected to a diagnostic catheter, or via syringe connected to an intervening manifold where contrast and saline can be drawn in and mixed before injection (Figure 4.1).

Power Injection: POWER is the key word here. This method requires specialized, automated injectors that deliver controlled amounts of

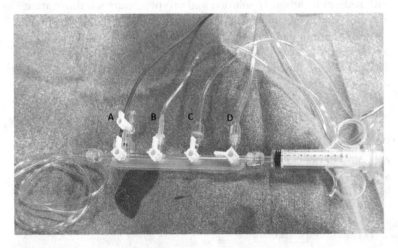

Figure 4.1 Manual contrast injection system with manifold. Manifold system includes connection ports for a pressure transducer for continuous intra-arterial pressure monitoring (A), pressurized saline (B), contrast (C), and a waste reservoir (D). (Helpful hint: The ports should be ordered so the least dangerous is farthest from the patient!)

Table 4.3 Guidelines for Contrast Power Injection by Vascular Bed

	Type of Catheter	Pressure (psi)	Rate of Rise (s)	Rate (mL/s)	Total Volume (mL)
Aortic arch	Flush	600–900	0.1	15	25–30
Carotid	End hole	300–500	0.7	3–5	6–10
Subclavian/brachial segments	End hole	300–500	0.7	3–5	6–10
Abdominal aorta	Flush	600–900	0.1	10	20–25
Superior mesenteric/celiac artery	End hole	200–500	1.0	3	6–20
Renal	End hole	200–500	1.0	3	6
Pelvic vessels	Flush	600	0.1	5–10	10–20
Infra-inguinal segments	End hole	300–500	0.7	3–5	6–10

contrast agent (5–40 mL) at selected pressures (400–1200 psi), best for imaging of large vessels (e.g., aorto-iliac) or large vascular territories (e.g., multi-segment single-run imaging of aorta to pedal vessels). In operating power injection equipment, multiple parameters of contrast delivery can be modulated (e.g., pressure rise, peak pressure, injection rate, injection delay, etc.), but contrast injection rate (mL/s) and total contrast volume delivered (mL per injection) are most frequently adjusted; common lingo in requesting injection settings is along the lines of "10 for 20, please," meaning setting the injector to deliver 10 mL/s of contrast for a total of 20 mL in total (see Table 4.3 for common settings for various endovascular imaging procedures) (8).

Carbon Dioxide (CO_2) Angiography: *The* alternative, although rarely used. When iodinated contrast agents cannot be safely used, intravascular administration of CO_2 gas as contrast can be used to perform angiographic imaging. Unlike iodinated agents, CO_2 functions to displace flowing blood, rather than mixing with it, to significantly reduce the amount of X-ray attenuation within the blood vessel lumen. Therefore, it serves as a **negative** contrast agent, making the vasculature appear lighter than the surrounding tissues. Despite its availability and use, image quality with CO_2 angiography is inferior to that of iodinated contrast, thus it is rarely used. When it is employed, CO_2 angiography is performed with a hand-injection system as seen in Figure 4.2.

Contraindications

Due to the risk of gas embolism, CO_2 absolutely cannot be used for any intra-arterial imaging **above** the diaphragm (9).

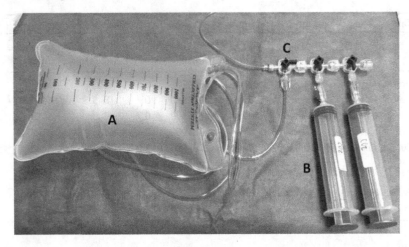

Figure 4.2 Common injection setup for CO_2 angiography. (A) A reservoir bag filled with CO_2 from wall port or gas tank via connected two-way stopcock to the delivery circuit. (B) Luer lock syringe (two in tandem in this manifold), which can be filled with CO_2 for injection via connected diagnostic catheter. (C) Intervening three-way stopcock and tubing system to modulate flow of CO_2 and ensure no introduction of air into the system.

Adverse Effects (9)

- Non-serious – Transient nausea, abdominal discomfort, leg cramping/pain.
- Serious/lethal – Air contamination of injectate due to defects in delivery system and subsequent air embolism, aortic vapor lock (occurs due to equilibration of CO_2 within the vasculature with non-soluble gases in the blood [e.g., N_2 and O_2], resulting in pockets of retained gaseous CO_2 that can cause mechanical obstruction of blood flow to visceral or peripheral vessels).

Key Points

- Iodinated contrast agents are utilized for angiographic imaging due to their ability to convey a vastly different degree of X-ray attenuation to the intravascular space.
- Iodinated agents carry with them the possibility of allergic reactions, contrast-induced nephropathy, and hyperthyroidism. Therefore, their use should be carefully evaluated in patients with documented severe allergic reactions, pre-existing renal dysfunction, or various thyroid conditions.

- Manual injection and power injection are the two main methods of contrast delivery for angiography. Manual injection is often used for medium-small vessels and can be accomplished with simple equipment, or slightly more complex manifold systems. Power injection delivers larger contrast volumes at high pressures and is most often employed for imaging larger vessels or large vascular beds. Learning how to assemble and operate this equipment is essential to performing high-quality angiographic imaging.
- CO_2 is a safe alternative to iodinated contrast agents, although intra-arterial administration above the diaphragm cannot be performed. This is used in some patients with CKD or severe contrast allergy. Severe complications of using this agent include gas embolism due to air contamination within the delivery system and aortic vapor lock. This imaging is inferior to iodinated agents.

References

1. Moresco KP, Patel N, Johnson MS, Trobridge D, Bergan KA, Lalka SG. Accuracy of CO_2 angiography in vessel diameter assessment: a comparative study of CO_2 versus iodinated contrast material in an aortoiliac flow model 1. J Vasc Interv Radiol. 2000;11(4):437–444.
2. Ali F, Mangi MA, Rehman H, Kaluski E. Use of carbon dioxide as an intravascular contrast agent: a review of current literature. World J Cardiol. 2017;9(9):715–722.
3. Bottinor W, Polkampally P. Adverse reactions to iodinated contrast media. Int J Angiol. 2013;22(3):149–153.
4. Mario S, Aberer W, Brockow K, Celik GE. Controversies in drug allergy: radiographic contrast media. J Allergy Clin Immunol Pract [Internet]. 2019;7(1):61–65. Available from: https://doi.org/10.1016/j.jaip.2018.06.030
5. Moriarity AK, Langer JM. Safe use of contrast media: what the radiologist needs to know. RadioGraphics. 2015;35(6):1738–1750.
6. Afshar AE. Prevention of contrast and radiation injury during coronary angiography and percutaneous coronary intervention. Curr Treat Option sin Cardiovasc Med. 2018;20(4):32.
7. Weisbord S, Gallagher M, Jneid H, Garcia S, Cass A, Thwin S, et al. Outcomes after angiography with sodium bicarbonate and acetylcysteine. N Engl J Med. 2018;378(7):603–614.
8. Kelso R, Kashyap VS. General principles of sedation, angiography, and intravascular ultrasound. In: Chaikof EL, Cambria RP, editors. Atlas of Vascular Surgery and Endovascular Therapy: Anatomy and Technique. Philadelphia: Elsevier Saunders; 2014. p. 17–28.
9. Sharafuddin MJ, Marjan AE, City I. Current status of carbon dioxide angiography. J Vasc Surg [Internet]. 2019;66(2):618–637. Available from: http://dx.doi.org/10.1016/j.jvs.2017.03.446

CHAPTER 5

VASCULAR ACCESS AND SHEATHS

Ahmad Younes, Jun Li

KEYWORDS

vascular access, sheath

LEARNING OBJECTIVES

- Understand the safe and effective way of various vascular access techniques
- Understand the potential access site complications and strategies to handle them
- Apply this safe skill set into alternative access sites when needed
- Recognize various sheath properties and sizing

Ensuring safe and efficient vascular access is a key element for successful endovascular intervention. The most frequent complications occurring during endovascular intervention are access site related (1–3). Access to an artery or vein can be obtained via percutaneous or open surgical approach. Compared with open surgical access, percutaneous access decreases wound complications with the trade-off of potentially less definitive hemostasis if not performed by skilled operators. Implementation of ultrasound (US) guidance for percutaneous access has reduced time to access and decreased complication rates.

Technique for Percutaneous Blood Vessel Access

In the most common technique (known as the modified Seldinger technique), the blood vessel is accessed with a hollow needle. After ensuring adequate position and blood return, a wire is thread into the vessel lumen, with care taken not to dissect the arterial walls (Figure 5.1). The original Seldinger technique was "modified" to avoid posterior wall penetration to prevent bleeding from the additional back wall through-and-through puncture (4). The course of the wire is confirmed using fluoroscopy, and subsequently a sheath or a catheter is advanced over the wire into the vessel. In our practice, we typically obtain access with a 21-gauge micropuncture kit and 0.018" access wire, with subsequent escalation to a larger sheath. This minimizes needle trauma and provides the opportunity to abort with less consequences should the access site be unfavorable.

Common Femoral Artery Access

Retrograde common femoral artery (CFA) remains the most conventional access site utilized for peripheral interventions (e.g., cerebrovascular, visceral, lower extremity) due to accompanying equipment lengths and amount of support afforded for interventions (1). A multimodality technique, combining anatomical assessment with imaging correlates, will minimize adverse outcomes (5). Correct identification of the overlying anatomical landmarks is the initial step.

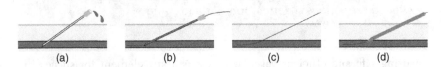

(a)	(b)	(c)	(d)

Figure 5.1 Modified Seldinger technique. (a) Access into the artery with a hollow needle. (b) While the needle is flattened to avoid dissecting the posterior wall, a wire is inserted carefully. (If the operator meets resistance as the wire exits the needle, it suggests that the wire is inside a dissection plane, in which case the needle should be repositioned slightly to allow entry into the true lumen. This may entail either negative tension backward, advancing forward, tilting of the needle either medially or laterally, or seldom rotation of the needle to allow a different interaction with the tip as the wire exits.) (c) Once the wire is in the true lumen of the vessel, the needle is withdrawn with pressure held over the site. (d) Either a sheath or microcatheter is inserted over the wire to secure the access.

One should begin by identifying the femoral triangle, which is defined by the following:

- The inguinal ligament superiorly (between the anterior superior iliac spine [ASIS] and pubic tubercle)
- The sartorius muscle laterally
- The adductor longus muscle medially

The femoral artery is encompassed within the femoral sheath in this triangle, along with the femoral vein and inguinal lymph nodes. The second important anatomical structure to identify is the femoral head, as it provides a hard surface for compression of the femoral artery when manual hemostasis is required at case completion and sheath removal (Figure 5.2A). The inguinal crease is not a reliable indicator of the most appropriate puncture site because of wide anatomical variations (6). This may be the most common technical error in femoral artery and venous access. In the obese population, the soft tissue may need to be retracted cephalad to allow proper access. Once the anatomical landmarks have been identified, one can then utilize fluoroscopic and/or US guidance to ensure identification of the correct puncture site.

Fluoroscopic Guidance: Typically, our practice is to place a hemostatic clamp at the inferior border of the femoral head for visualization fluoroscopically (Figure 5.2B). The ideal entry point is distal to the inferior epigastric artery (IEA) and proximal to the bifurcation into superficial femoral artery (SFA) and profunda femoris artery (PFA). In the majority of patients, the inferior loop of the IEA is above the middle of the femoral head. There is more variation on the level of the bifurcation of SFA and PFA, though it is distal to the lower quarter of the femoral head in approximately 85% of patients (7). To optimize the chances of access within the target zone, we recommend aiming for needle entry into the artery within the mid to lower one third of the femoral head (Figure 5.2C–E).

US Guidance: US allows direct visualization of the femoral bifurcation (Figure 5.3) to ensure puncture in the CFA, an anterior wall stick, and avoidance of calcification. Frequency probes greater than 7 MHz are typically used for accessing superficial arteries, although probes with less than 7 MHz transducers are suitable for deeper structures as well (e.g., distal SFA). Smaller and more superficial vessels, such as the radial and pedal arteries, are best visualized with a hockey stick linear array transducer (13–18 MHz) with its slimmer profile and smaller footprint.

Once the target vessel is identified under US, the probe is fixed in the desired location. After local anesthesia, a needle is advanced at 45 degrees angulation into the direction of the probe (Figure 5.2C) (8). For deeper vasculature structures, the skin entry point is further away from the probe,

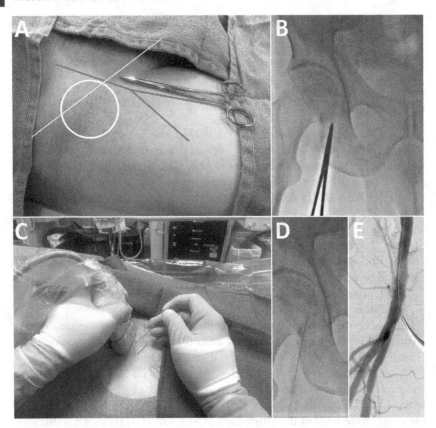

Figure 5.2 The anatomy of the groin (A) should be assessed as the first step. The femoral head (circle) should be identified, as well as the point of maximal pulsation atop the femoral head. The inguinal ligament (light gray) is oftentimes proximal to where the anatomical crease is. We oftentimes place a hemostat at the mid to lower edge of the femoral head to mark the anticipated entry site (B). US guidance (C) is useful to ensure puncture into the CFA, to avoid access into the SFA or PFA, and to circumvent areas with a high degree of anterior calcium. Note the relationship of the angle of the needle with the US probe, taking into account the body habitus of the patient. For a patient with a larger habitus, one should utilize either a steeper angulation for access, or enter the skin at a more distal point, so as to traverse the necessary soft tissue to reach the artery at the location of insonation. Fluoroscopic confirmation (D) of the puncture site at the mid to lower third of the femoral head using a micropuncture kit prior to upsizing to a larger sheath will minimize bleeding, in the event that a redo puncture is needed. Femoral angiogram (E) should be performed prior to the conclusion of the case to evaluate for vessel sizing, location of access, and presence of CFA disease to determine candidacy for closure device. (Abbreviations: *CFA*, common femoral artery; *PFA*, profunda femoris artery; *SFA*, superficial femoral artery.)

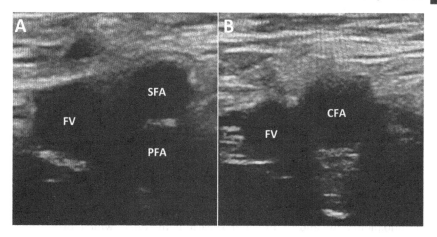

Figure 5.3 With direct visualization using a US probe, the bifurcation of the SFA and PFA (A) can be easily identified, with a puncture into the CFA (B). This minimizes adverse events such as bleeding and pseudoaneurysms, while also optimizing the chances of using a closure device at the conclusion of the case to achieve hemostasis. (Abbreviations: *CFA*, common femoral artery; *FV*, femoral vein; *PFA*, profunda femoris artery; *SFA*, superficial femoral artery.)

as opposed to more superficial structures, whereby the skin entry point is oftentimes abutting the probe. Conversely, for larger habitus patients with very deep CFA, one may need to adjust the angulation of the needle to 60–80 degrees to ensure needle length is sufficient to allow puncture into the artery. We often have an assistant alert the primary operator of blood return to prevent posterior wall penetration.

Radial Artery Access

Access via the radial artery remains popular for both peripheral (e.g., visceral, renal, proximal femoral, iliac, subclavian/innominate, carotid) and coronary interventions. For access, the arm is positioned and secured in the supine position, with the thumb extended. Using either the traditional or modified Seldinger technique, the radial artery is accessed at 45 degrees angulation and the wire is advanced slowly to avoid dissection. Some operators prefer the use of an angiocath for access of the radial artery. In patients with small radial arteries, subcutaneous nitroglycerin and use of US may be helpful. Anticoagulation should be administered immediately after obtaining access to reduce the risk of thrombosis and occlusion. We typically administer 100 units of heparin per kilogram of body weight for interventional procedures, and half-dose (50 units/kg) for diagnostic imaging only.

An important consideration in utilization of the radial artery is the distance anticipated to the target lesion. The left arm provides a shorter distance needed to travel to reach the descending aorta and avoids traversing across the great vessels, although the right arm is more ergonomic for most interventionalists.

Brachial Artery Access

Access via the brachial artery is useful for many of the same interventions in which radial access is used (peripheral and coronary), with the benefit of more proximal access for greater stability in lesion crossing and device delivery. It should be noted that while percutaneous access can be obtained via the brachial artery, it comes with significant risks of brachial artery thrombosis, pseudoaneurysm, and/or brachial sheath hematoma, which oftentimes require open surgical repair. In vascular surgery practices, it is common for access at this site to be obtained via open surgical exposure to allow primary arteriotomy closure and definitive hemostasis (9, 10)

For percutaneous access, the arm is positioned in an extended fashion and secured in the supine position. Access over the olecranon is crucial to allow hemostasis during manual compression. We recommend first identifying the underlying bone, then palpating the artery for the point of maximal impulse. US guidance with micropuncture access needle is strongly recommended to minimize inadvertent access of adjacent venous structures and/or injury to the median nerve. Front wall puncture only with the modified Seldinger technique is ideal in this space. Anticoagulation immediately after obtaining access is necessary to reduce the risk of thrombosis.

Alternative Access Sites

Current era endovascular interventions require one to be facile in alternative access sites, including antegrade femoral, distal SFA, tibial, and pedal vessels. Each of these sites can be tailored to different revascularization strategies. Distal SFA, tibial, and pedal access are typically used for retrograde crossing of long segment chronic total occlusions, though may occasionally be necessary for equipment delivery as well. These are further detailed below.

Antegrade Femoral Artery Access: In planned tibial and pedal revascularization, antegrade femoral access site will provide better support and delivery of wires and interventional equipment. This may be particularly useful in patients who have tortuous iliac arteries, extreme angulation of the iliac bifurcation, are very tall, or have complex tibial disease requiring advanced crossing techniques. Importantly, one must be certain that inflow disease has been excluded prior to attempting antegrade access to ensure adequate flow into the tibial arteries after intervention.

The abdominal wall is retracted cephalad and access into the CFA is obtained with a standard 18-gauge access needle at approximately 75–85 degrees angulation, either under fluoroscopic or US guidance. Once bleed back is noted, the angulation of the needle is lowered, and a Versacore (Abbott Vascular) or Wholey (Medtronic) wire is advanced. Targeting the needle towards the medial aspect of the patient will increase the chances of wiring the SFA successfully, rather than the PFA. If the wire travels into the PFA, and the arteriotomy site is certain to be within the CFA, one may attempt withdrawing the wire and carefully attempting to engage the SFA under fluoroscopic guidance. However, this maneuver may result in loss of access, so alternatively, one may place a 5Fr 10-cm introducer sheath into the PFA. Under fluoroscopic monitoring, the sheath is slowly withdrawn into the CFA while maintaining the Versacore or Wholey wire position in the PFA. As the sheath is placed into the CFA, one may then utilize a 0.035″ stiff angled Glidewire (Terumo) to engage the SFA under fluoroscopic guidance. The PFA wire is removed, and the dilator is placed onto the stiff angled Glidewire to advance the sheath into the SFA.

Distal Femoral Access: For long, occlusive segments in the SFA, a retrograde approach into the distal SFA may be necessary as an adjunctive technique to allow successful recanalization. We typically avoid popliteal access, as it requires the patient to be prone. In patients who require distal femoral access, the leg may be externally rotated slightly, with the image intensifier positioned in a shallow contralateral oblique view (approximately 10–20 degrees) to decrease parallax of the artery. In highly calcified vessels or those with a previously placed stent, fluoroscopic guidance without contrast is oftentimes sufficient to obtain access. In the absence of this, we recommend injection of contrast as access is being obtained to allow for visualization of the vessel. An 18-gauge needle is utilized, followed by careful advancement of a stiff angled Glidewire (Terumo). One should be careful not to shear the wire during attempted advancement and retraction. A contralateral view may be necessary to assess the depth of the needle in relation to the vessel itself prior to advancement of the wire. Following wire advancement, we typically use a sheathless approach with a bareback microcatheter as support for crossing the occluded segment. With microcatheter access only, manual compression or intraarterial balloon tamponade at the site of entry will suffice for hemostasis during the procedure. However, if a sheath is used retrograde into the distal SFA, hemostasis can be achieved with manual extrinsic compression after the activated clotting time is within range (<170 seconds).

Pedal Access: Retrograde tibial and pedal access techniques are vital for a dedicated limb-salvage specialist, as these alternative access sites are oftentimes necessary as adjunctive techniques for crossing chronic total occlusions. More superficial vessels, such as the dorsalis pedis and distal posterior tibial artery, can be accessed using a hockey stick linear array probe. Deeper structures, such as the distal peroneal artery and proximal anterior tibial artery, may be better visualized with fluoroscopic guidance utilizing calcium as guidance or concomitant antegrade contrast injection. In the tibial arteries, oftentimes a 0.014″ or 0.018″ system is sufficient to traverse the occlusive segments. Given this, and to limit trauma to the target vessel, we typically forgo sheath insertion into the tibials and utilize a microcatheter for support only. In some circumstances, where a 0.035″ system is desired (e.g., to traverse a recalcitrant SFA and popliteal occlusion), upsizing to a short 4Fr pedal sheath may be necessary to allow passage of a larger support catheter. Ensuring hemostasis of the retrograde site prior to transfer out of the catheterization laboratory or angiography suite is essential to prevent any adverse outcomes.

Complications

It is important to be familiar with potential access site complications and their management.

Table 5.1 Common Target Access Vessels, Complications, and Management.

Target Access Vessel	Complication	Management
Brachial artery	Bleeding, hematoma, nerve damage	Open surgical decompression and repair
Radial artery	Spasm (most frequent, 6–10% of patients) (11)	Reduce incidence with pre-procedural sedation, hydrophilic sheaths, intraarterial vasodilators after sheath insertion* If there is significant traction on the sheath during removal, do not aggressively pull, as it may result in arterial avulsion. Sedation and maximized vasodilation is necessary. In difficult to sedate patients, intubation and general anesthesia may be necessary in the very extreme cases.
	Occlusion (second most frequent, 3–10% asymptomatic, 0.3% asymptomatic)**	Reduce incidence with small sheaths, intra-procedural heparin, and post-procedural "patent hemostasis" with band devices. For symptomatic RAO, compression of ulnar artery to improve collaterals and administration of systemic anticoagulation will be helpful. Radial artery endovascular recanalization or surgery may be rarely be needed to help restore flow

(Continued)

Target Access Vessel	Complication	Management
Radial artery (Continued)	Perforation (uncommon, 0.04%),	Tamponade with catheter or sheath itself (1%). Forearm compartment syndrome is rare but requires surgery. Inflate a blood pressure cuff over the perforation with maintained inflation 10–15 mmHg above the systolic blood pressure for at least 15 minutes at a time may stop any active bleeding. Reverse anticoagulation. Repeat angiogram or operate if necessary
Femoral artery	Thrombosis	There is a higher risk of complication using a percutaneous closure device with antegrade compared with traditional retrograde deployment (12)
	Bleeding, groin and retroperitoneal hematomas	Continued manual pressure for local groin bleeding. If there is a high index of suspicion for retroperitoneal bleeding, one may consider emergency relook angiogram +/- surgery. CT scan may be helpful in a more clinically stable patient with a lower clinical suspicion. covered stent placement for retroperitoneal bleeding ± surgical repair

* Cocktail typically consists of nitroglycerin (100–200 µg) ± calcium channel blockers (verapamil 2.5–5 mg, diltiazem 2.5–5 mg, or nicardipine 250–500 µg); vasoactive medications should be utilized with caution in patients with cardiogenic shock, severely reduced ejection fraction, or severe aortic stenosis (13).

** The most current multi-societal recommendations do not advise routine pre-procedural testing for collateral hand circulation (Allen or Barbeau), as an abnormal test should not prohibit transradial access (14).

Sheaths

After initial access to a vessel is obtained, it must be maintained without continuous bleeding from the access hole. This is made possible with the use of hemostatic sheaths through which all wires, catheters, and interventional devices are inserted into a vessel. Such sheaths are generally constructed

Table 5.2 Available Reinforced Sheaths from Various Vendors, with Available Sizes and Lengths

	Company	Size (Fr)	Length (cm)	Guidewire Compatibility (inch)	Tip Shape	Radiopaque Tip	Hydrophilic Coating
Fortress	Biotronik	4, 5, 6	45/100	0.035	Straight, curved	Yes	No
Flexor: Ansel	Cook Medical	4–9	45, 55, 90, 110	0.018 (4.5 Fr only), 0.038	Straight, curved, multipurpose	Yes	Yes
Flexor: Ansel High Flex	Cook Medical	4–8, 10,12	45, 55, 70	0.035	Straight, multipurpose	Yes	Yes
Flexor: Balkin	Cook Medical	5.5–8	40,45	0.038	Curved	Yes	Both available
Flexor: Shuttle Family	Cook Medical	4–8	80, 90, 110	0.018 (4.5 Fr only), 0.038	Straight	Yes	Yes
Flexor: Standard	Cook Medical	5–10, 12	13, 30, 40, 45, 80, 90	0.038	Straight	Yes	No
The Sheath	Medtronic	7–8	55	0.038	Straight	Yes	No
AXS Infinity LS	Stryker	8	70, 80, 90	0.035, 0.038	Straight	Yes	Yes
Super Arrow-Flex Sheath	Teleflex	5–11	11–100	0.035	Straight, curved	Yes	Yes
Pinnacle Destination Guiding Sheath	Terumo	5, 6, 7, 8	45, 65, 90	0.038	Straight, multipurpose, hockey stick, renal double curve, LIMA	Yes	Yes
R2P Destination Slender Guiding Sheath	Terumo	6	119, 149, 200	0.038	Straight	Yes	Yes

Abbreviations: Fr, French; LIMA, left internal mammary artery.

as a hollow catheter, which is capped by an apparatus containing an in-line hemostatic valve and a perpendicularly oriented side port with stopcock for flushes and contrast injection.

For the majority of interventions, both coronary and peripheral, we typically first obtain access with a shorter and smaller sheath (e.g., 5Fr 10-cm sheath) to perform our angiograms with diagnostic catheters. After the lesion of interest is identified, we then upsize to a larger and longer sheath for a more direct engagement into the target vessel (periphery or carotids) or exchange for guiding catheters (guides) (coronary, intra-abdominal vessels). The French size on sheaths refers to the inner diameter (ID), as opposed to the outer diameter (OD), when referencing catheters and guides (15). For example, a 6Fr sheath will have an ID of 2.2 mm and an OD of 2.8 mm, whereas a 6Fr catheter may have an ID of 1.37 mm and an OD of 2.0 mm. With the larger overall ID, sheaths allow for more versatility in equipment delivery; most peripheral interventions are performed through long sheaths to take advantage of this characteristic.

Given anatomical variations in coronary and intra-abdominal vessels, guides are oftentimes utilized to provide the versatility to engage these vessels. Table 5.2 lists a sampling of reinforced sheaths available; specific ID and OD vary by manufacturer.

Summary

Instrumental in the success of an endovascular intervention is access planning and execution. Safe and consistent technique will minimize adverse access site-related events. Versatility with both fluoroscopic and US guidance will help minimize radiation and contrast exposure. Sheaths, diagnostic catheters, and guiding catheters are merely the starting equipment that the endovascular interventionalist ought to be well acquainted with. Interventional wires and support catheters are discussed in detail in the following chapters.

Key Points
- Careful planning and safe execution of vascular access is a critical component of the endovascular procedural success.
- Adjunctive imaging with US guidance will minimize adverse events associated with access.
- A proper understanding of sheath sizing and properties as well as equipment sizes is required prior to endovascular procedures.

References

1. Ortiz D, Jahangir A, Singh M, Allaqaband S, Mewissen M. Access site complications after peripheral vascular interventions: incidence, predictors, and outcomes. Circ Cardiovasc Interv. 2014;7(6):821–828.
2. Krajcer Z, Howell M. Update on endovascular treatment of peripheral vascular disease. Texas Hear Inst J. 2000;27(4):369–385.
3. Kasapis C, Gurm HS, Chetcuti SJ, Munir K, Luciano A, Smith D, et al. Defining the optimal degree of heparin anticoagulation for peripheral vascular interventions. Circ Cardiovasc Interv. 2010;3(6):593–601.
4. Seldinger SI. Catheter replacement of the needle in percutaneous arteriography: a new technique. Acta Radiol. 1953;39(5):368–376.
5. Lo RC, Fokkema MTM, Curran T, Darling J, Hamdan AD, Wyers M, et al. Routine use of ultrasound-guided access reduces access site-related complications after lower extremity percutaneous revascularization. J Vasc Surg. [Internet]. 2012;61(2):405–412. Available from: http://dx.doi.org/10.1016/j.jvs.2014.07.099
6. Grier D, Hartnell G. Percutaneous femoral artery puncture: practice and anatomy. Br J Radiol. 1990;63(752):602–604.
7. Ahn H, Lee H, Lee H, Yang J, Yi J, Lee I. Assessment of the optimal site of femoral artery puncture and angiographic anatomical study of the common femoral artery. J Korean Neurosurg Soc. 2014;56(2):91–97.
8. Sandoval Y, Burke MN, Lobo AS, Lips DL, Seto AH, Chavez I, et al. Contemporary arterial access in the cardiac catheterization laboratory. J Am Coll Cardiol Cardiovasc Interv. 2017;10(22):2233–2241.
9. Alvarez-Tostado JA, Moise MA, Bena JF, Pavkov ML, Greenberg RK, Clair DG, et al. The brachial artery: a critical access for endovascular procedures. J Vasc Surg. 2009;49(2):378–385.
10. Madden NJ, Calligaro KD, Zheng H, Troutman DA, Dougherty MJ. Outcomes of brachial artery access for endovascular interventions. Ann Vasc Surg. 2019;56:81–86.
11. Patel T, Shah S, Sanghvi K, Pancholy S. Management of radial and brachial artery perforations during transradial procedures – a practical approach. J Invasive Cardiol. 2009;21(10):544–547.
12. Barbetta I, van den Berg JC. Access and hemostasis: femoral and popliteal approaches and closure devices – why, what, when, and how? Semin Intervent Radiol. 2014;31(4):353–360.
13. Coppola J, Patel T, Kwan T, Sanghvi K, Srivastava S, Shah S, et al. Nitroglycerin, nitroprusside, or both, in preventing radial artery spasm during transradial artery catheterization. J Invasive Cardiol. 2006;18(4):155–158.
14. Mason PJ, Shah B, Tamis-Holland JE, Bittl JA, Cohen MG, Safirstein J, et al. An update on radial artery access and best practices for transradial coronary angiography and intervention in acute coronary syndrome. Circ Cardiovasc Interv. 2018;11(9):1–21.
15. From AM, Gulati R, Prasad A, Rihal CS. Sheathless transradial intervention using standard guide catheters. Catheter Cardiovasc Interv. 2010;76(7):911–916.

CHAPTER 6

GUIDEWIRES

Justin A. Smith, Ravi N. Ambani, Karem C. Harth

KEYWORDS

guidewire, working wire, interventional wire

LEARNING OBJECTIVES

- Understand the role that guidewires play in the delivery of endovascular devices and therapies
- Understand the basic anatomy of a guidewire
  - Conceptualize how modulating different core, tip, body, and coating construction parameters affects wire performance
- Develop a fundamental understanding of wire performance characteristics and common wires that embody desired characteristics

The delivery of catheters or endovascular devices for angiography and intervention requires that a path to their target vessel be established by a wire. The expansion of endovascular technology has included a commensurate growth in the available wires. Unique properties of these wires include various combinations of tip and body construction, sizes, and coatings that offer performance advantages in navigating different vascular beds, crossing lesions and supporting therapeutic devices. Wires can be divided into four basic groups:

1. **Access Wires:** These are short, stiff wires that allow access/safe placement of a sheath (i.e., often packed with sheath kit, micro-puncture access kit, Cope wire).

2. **Traditional Guidewire:** A guidewire will allow us to navigate across the vessel of interest and is soft with a floppy tip to avoid vessel injury (i.e., standard J-wire, Bentson wire).

3. **Support ("Working") Wires:** These wires are stiff wires, built to provide the support necessary to deliver an endovascular device (i.e., Rosen, Amplatz, Lunderquist).

4. **Specialty Wires:** These wires have a coating or have hybrid construction for a specific application (i.e., hydrophilic Glidewire, V18 wire with hydrophilic tip and stiff body).

This chapter will focus on both aspects of the clinical use of guidewires, as well as finer point of their construction to provide a foundation to understand their properties and thus their specific functions. While a grasp of these concepts of use, and technical details, is helpful, equally important is gaining real-world experience with a particular wire until you understand how it will behave in a vessel or lesion. With experience, the operator can utilize visual *and* tactile feedback from the wire to successfully perform an endovascular procedure.

Wire Anatomy

A wire has four components: core, tip, body, and coating.

Core: The core runs the entire length of the wire, providing internal structure and support to both the shaft and the tip (Figure 6.1). The shaft will carry catheters and devices along its length while the tip is designed for vessel navigation and lesion crossing (1). The construction of the core

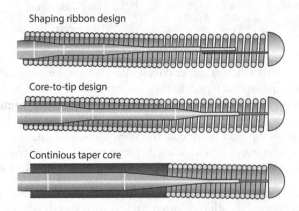

Shaping ribbon design

Core-to-tip design

Continious taper core

Figure 6.1 Guidewire core and tip constructions.

can be fairly complex in order to allow its functions to change along the wire's length. Components that contribute to the overall construct of the core include: material, diameter, the degree of taper, and the presence of grinds (Figure 6.1).

Core Material: Stainless steel and nitinol are the primary materials found in the core of wires. Stainless steel is generally stiffer, providing the user with greater ability to steer the guidewire tip and superior support, while flexible enough to navigate tortuous vessels; this material also retains its shape better, conveying greater durability (2). Stainless steel can generally be found in the cores of support/working wires (e.g., Amplatz, Lunderquist) used to carry large endografts (thoracic endovascular aortic repair [TEVAR], endovascular aneurysm repair [EVAR]) where a stiff guide is paramount to ensuring these devices track safely and reliably into place. Nitinol is known for being malleable and highly flexible. Malleability allows better navigation along more tortuous vessels while flexibility allows it to be resistant to kinking, which would prevent further passage down a vessel (2). Such nitinol cores are useful in specialty wires used to navigate tortuous vessels, or cross-complex lesions, conveying good support with the flexibility to track and cross, establishing initial access to be used for wire exchange or device delivery. Wire cores can be either homogenous in their material construction or heterogeneous with transitions from proximal to distal (usually stainless steel at the shaft and nitinol at the tip).

Core Diameter: The strength and support of wires is directly proportional to core diameter (strength and support α radius cubed [radius^4]). Thus, a 0.035″ diameter wire provides more strength and support compared with a 0.014″ wire of similar construction.

Core Taper and Grind: The core material of a wire tip is usually tapered to narrow its diameter distally and provide a tip that flexes and bends at its very end (strength α radius^4) to help navigate vessel turns and find the channels across lesions. This taper can be continuous, occurring in a steep or gradual manner toward the wire tip, or it can be interrupted by areas of constant diameter (grinds) that maintain the wire tip strength closer to the wire end (Figure 6.1). Short/abrupt tapers produce a wire tip that provides greater support, but may have a tendency to prolapse into adjacent vessels. Where the very distal tip is flexible and will track nicely into branches, it is followed by the remainder of the wire that quickly stiffens and may pull the tip out of these branches. Longer tapers produce wire tips with less support but better ability to track farther into target vessels before stiffer wire portions have the chance to cause any prolapsing effect (Figure 6.2). Wire tips can vary in the presence, number, length, and position of core grinds (3).

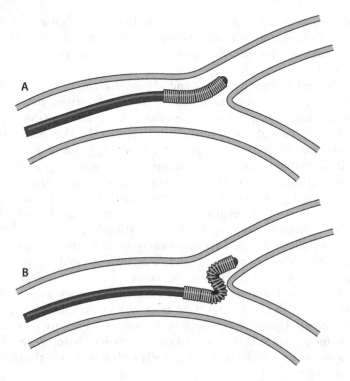

Figure 6.2 (A) Successful wire tacking into a branch vessel using a guidewire with a longer taper or more numerous/longer grinds. (B) Guidewire prolapse resulting in less effective tracking in a guidewire with a short taper or fewer/shorter/absent grinds.

Tip: Tips come in two major styles: core-to-tip and shaping ribbon (Figure 6.1). Core-to-tip wires connect their tip core to the very end of the wire, allowing better transmission of force from the operator to the wire tip, and thus better steering and tactile feedback (the ability of the user to sense resistance to or passage of the wire tip from the opposite end). Such a design can be useful in specialty chronic total occlusion (CTO) wires used to drill through hard, calcified occlusive lesions to establish initial access across them. On the other hand, the shaping ribbon design is built to be soft and flexible as the core does not connect with the wire tip, thus reducing support of the tip from the core and is more easily deflected. This can be useful for probing lesions to find any natural channels that can be leveraged for an easier and less traumatic crossing of complex occlusions/stenoses. Additionally, the shaping ribbon design allows the interventionalist to manually bend or shape the end of the wire to produce a wire with a custom tip curve that can be directed by twisting the wire, thus steering it to direct the tip for selecting branch vessels as the wire is advanced (2).

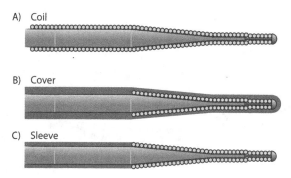

A) Coil

B) Cover

C) Sleeve

Figure 6.3 Guidewire body styles. (A) Coil body style consisting of wound coil covering from shaft to tip without additional coatings. (B) Cover body style in which the entire wire is coated in polymer, including distal coils that support the more flexible tip. (C) Sleeve body style with a discrete transition where the shaft, coated in polymer, meets and uncoated coil-wound tip.

Body: The body is the structure that surrounds the wire core and serves to modify wire friction, tactile feedback, as well as deformability and shape retention of the tip. Spring coils, covers, and sleeves are the general classes of body styles (Figure 6.3). Spring coils serve to maintain guidewire shape, supporting the shaft and allowing the distal end to recoil back to its baseline shape. Covers consist of a polymer/plastic coating of the entire wire with coils contained within the distal end. The coatings provide friction-modulating capabilities (discussed below), while allowing some recoil toward the more flexible tip. Last, sleeves are a hybrid body, composed of coil and cover technology. The distal end (coil) is surrounded by bare coils to provide an end with greater tactile feedback with resistance to kinking/deformation. The proximal end (cover) is a coated shaft to provide various degrees of tracking (1).

Coating: The addition of polymers/plastics to the wires alter their friction along the vessel wall as well as the tactile feedback to the user. In general, hydrophilic coatings convey a lubricity (felt as a gel-like slippery character) to the wire when wet, giving it enhanced maneuverability, which is important in tortuous anatomy. Unfortunately, this comes at the expense of less tactile feedback as the wire will slip through the vessel and slip through the operators hand when encountering resistance (such wires may require the use of a torque device screwed onto the wire to provide a secure handle from which to twist and advance the wire against resistance) (Figure 6.4). Conversely, hydrophobic coatings allow for greater tactile feedback but reduced ease in tracking through tortuous vessels due to the resistance from friction with the vessel wall (1, 2).

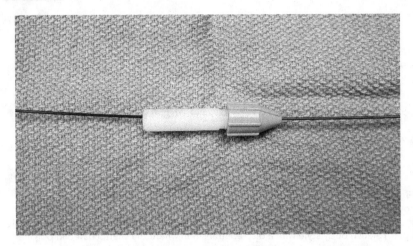

Figure 6.4 Torque device secured to a hydrophilic wire for easier manipulation.

Wire Parameters

Dimensions: The two primary measurements for wires are length and diameter. While manufacturers produce wires of a variety of lengths typically ranging from 80 to 300 cm, there are a number of common lengths including 80, 150, 180, and 260 cm (Table 6.1) (4). More recently, advances in peripheral interventions with access sites in the radial artery have extended wire lengths as long as 450 cm. However, this group of wires is limited and still under development. Typically, wires 260 cm and greater in length are termed "exchange length" wires as they allow the interventionalist the ability to treat more distal disease from the access point while maintaining wire access. Externally (outside the body/

Table 6.1 Wire Lengths for Various Intervention Targets

Length (cm)	Interventions
<80	Initial vascular access, ipsilateral iliofemoral arteriography, ipsilateral dialysis access angiography and/or interventions (limited utility)
150–180	Aortoiliac, renal/mesenteric arteriography. Ipsilateral or contralateral iliac intervention from femoral access
180–260	Coronary angiography and interventions, carotid and arch arteriography, mesenteric and renal interventions, contralateral infra-inguinal interventions from femoral access
>260	Transfemoral carotid interventions, aortic stent-graft interventions, and tibial interventions

sheath), one can remove devices over the wire while having manual control of the wire at all times. A good rule of thumb is that delivery of an interventional device or catheter will require a wire a little more than twice the length of the distance from the access site to the vessel/lesion of interest so that the wire can reach this area, but the device may be loaded onto the back and advanced while maintaining manual wire control on either end. Wire diameters are measured in fractions of an inch, and come in standard measures of 0.014″, 0.018″, 0.035″, and 0.038″. Simply explained, larger diameter wires are stronger and bulkier, whereas smaller diameter wires are weaker and thinner. Within each of the wire diameters, there are the above core, tip, body, and coating adaptations that can exist to improve the wire design and provide options. The wire diameters are important to understand as the catheters and devices available for intervention are typically designed for a certain wire diameter support. In general, the larger diameter wires are appropriate for larger vessel interventions (iliacs, femoral, aorta). Smaller diameter wires are more appropriate for smaller vessel interventions (coronaries, tibials, carotids, mesenterics).

Performance Characteristics: The summation of guidewire core construction, tip design, body, and coatings all contribute to the overall performance exhibited by a wire. Table 6.2 outlines the various characteristics of a wire's performance, its definition, and some examples of wires that can provide these characteristics

Table 6.2 Performance Characteristics of Wires with Examples

Performance Characteristic	Definition	Examples
Trackability	Ability to guide the tip down a vessel regardless of anatomy (tortuosity)	Glidewire, Benson
Torqueability (pushability)	Ability to translate rotational forces at the operator end into rotation at the tip end of the wire	Steelcore, Glidewire Advantage, Stiff Glidewire
Flexibility	Ability to flex about the wire's longitudinal axis	Spartacore, Glidewire (Nonstiff), Benson
Crossability	Ability to cross a lesion with minimal resistance	Command 18, V18, V14, Gold Glidewire, Stiff Glidewire, Confianza, Journey
Supportability	Ability to facilitate passage of devices over the wire	Rosen, SV5, Grand Slam, Lunderquist, Glidewire Advantage
Penetrating power	[Tip load (g)*]/[tip area (in²)]	Confianza, Connect 250T, Command 18, V18

* Amount of force required to deflect a guidewire tip.

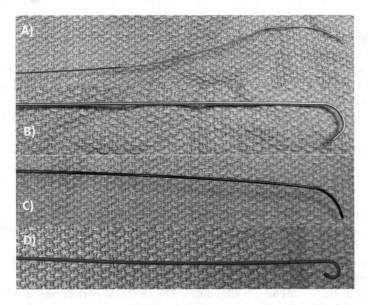

Figure 6.5 Guidewire examples. (A) Microwire (Cook Medical®). (B) J-wire. (C) Soft-angled Glidewire® (Terumo® Interventional Systems). (D) Rosen wire (Cook Medical®).

(see Figure 6.5 for images of several of these guidewires). These characteristics underlie how dynamic and variable wires can be, as a single wire can possess several notable performance characteristics to various degrees based on the combination of core design, tip design, coatings, and so forth, chosen to build that particular wire. Perhaps most important regarding these characteristics that an interventionalist really only gets a handle on them through trial and error, playing and experimenting with the wires they have available to them through the training years and throughout their professional practice.

Summary

This overview of wire technology is but a glimpse of a large area of science that is ever evolving. Understanding the basics can make an intervention more efficient and successful. Selection of a wire will depend on the access site location, vascular bed of interest, and complexity of intervention. Re-cannalizing an occluded vessel or deploying an aortic stent graft will require a very different wire selection compared with steering across a tortuous open vessel leading to the tibial arteries. It is important to consider that wires are not used in isolation, and understanding support catheters can further enhance the capabilities and strengths of your chosen wire.

Key Points

- Wires serve to establish access to vessels and lesions and allow the delivery and support of catheters for imaging and devices for intervention.
- Wire construction can be fairly complex, composed of a core, body, tip, and coating.
- Wire construct contributes to the performance and function of a wire.
- Selection of a wire will depend on the access site location, vascular bed of interest, and complexity of intervention.

References

1. Tóth GG, Yamane M, Heyndrickx GR. How to select a guidewire: technical features and key characteristics. Heart. 2015;101:645–652.
2. Walker BC. Guidewire selection for peripheral vascular interventions. Endovascular Today. 2013;80–83.
3. Gupta S. Guide catheters & guidewire: overview and case illustrations. In: Society for Cardiovascular Angioplasty and Interventions Fellows Course [Internet]. 2015. Available from: http://www.scai.org/Assets/31e9f931-160b-459c-9d7b-b6771621b642/635742456224670000/gupta-guidecatheters-and-guidewire-pdf
4. Schneider PA. Guidewire-catheter skills. Endovascular Skills. 3rd ed. Boca Raton, FL: Taylor & Francis Group; 2009. p. 57–61.

CATHETERS

Lisa Walker, Eric McLoney

KEYWORDS

catheter, flush, selective angiographic, microcatheter, guide catheter, support catheter

LEARNING OBJECTIVES

- To learn the fundamental concepts of catheters
- To understand the measurements of catheters
- To distinguish different types of catheters and their various purposes

Catheter selection is key to a successful interventional procedure. In the past, catheters were specially customized and hand-shaped for each patient. However, since the advancement of minimally invasive endovascular procedures, there is now a myriad of pre-shaped catheters by different companies. This chapter will discuss the fundamental concepts of catheters and their selection.

Catheter Characteristics

The characteristics of different catheters depend on the material, shape, size, length, and the presence of side holes. Catheters are made out of different materials including polyethylene, polyurethane, nylon, and Teflon (polytetrafluoroethylene) (1). Catheters can be braided to improve torque or can be coated with hydrophilic material for improved trackability (2).

Table 7.1 Catheter Measurements	
Outer diameter	French (Fr; 1Fr = 1/3 mm)
Inner diameter	Inches (in)
Length	Centimeters (cm)

Catheters are divided into three parts: hub, shaft, and tip. The hub is the proximal end of the catheter, and is the entry site for guidewires and contrast injection. The shaft of the catheter is variable in length, and length selection is determined by the type and location of the procedure. The tip of the catheter is the most varied portion of the catheter in its shape and functionality (1). The tip of the catheter can be either an end-hole catheter or a side-hole catheter. As the name suggests, end-hole catheters have one hole at the end; these are often selective catheters and are used for administration of contrast and embolic materials. Side-hole catheters have additional holes near the tip of the catheter and are the workhorse for diagnostic imaging of vessels and injection of contrast in larger volumes (3).

There are three key measurements to define catheters: outer diameter, inner diameter, and length. The outer diameter is measured in French size, and this determines which size vascular sheath will fit inside. The inner diameter is measured in inches and determines the luminal size and thereby which size wire or microcatheter will fit inside. The length of the catheter is measured in centimeters, and selection depends on the access site and target location (Table 7.1) (3). Typical catheter lengths are 65 cm for abdominal and pelvic procedures, 100 cm for thoracic procedures, and 120 cm for peripheral extremity procedures (1). The most commonly used catheter sizes are 4 and 5Fr. The flow rates for catheters are dependent on the catheter diameter, length, presence of side holes, and pressure rating. These are specified on the packaging.

Catheter Types

Nonselective Flush "Diagnostic" Catheters: These catheters have multiple side holes that allow for a large bolus of rapid contrast delivery and are ideal for aortography and venacavography. There are three main types (Figure 7.1):

1. **Pigtail Catheter:** This catheter has a characteristic "pigtail"-shaped loop at the end. The loop contains numerous side holes and an end hole. The pigtail catheter will straighten when a guidewire is advanced inside the catheter and forms when the guidewire is

Pigtail	Omni	Straight
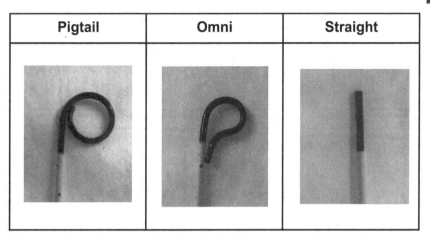		

Figure 7.1 Commonly used flush catheters.

withdrawn. Pigtail catheters come in a variety of diameters; however, the most commonly used are the 15-mm diameter ones.

2. **Omni Flush:** This catheter has a tight reverse curve and numerous side holes. It is often called a "shepherd's hook" catheter given its shape.

3. **Straight Flush:** This is a straight-shaped catheter with numerous side holes and an end hole. This catheter is used in vessels too small to accommodate a pigtail but has high flow, such as the iliac arteries.

Selective Catheters: This group of catheters has varied shaped tips for access to different vessels (2, 3). They can be ordered from simple, angled catheters to multi-angled, complex catheters (Figure 7.2):

1. **Single Angled Catheters**
   a. **Kumpe, Berenstein, Glide Catheter:** A variety of catheters exist with a simple angle at the end, which is variable in length.
   b. **Multipurpose Angled Catheter (MPA):** This catheter was designed to decrease the need of multiple different catheters. It has a single curve and, depending on the type, may have an end hole with or without side holes. It can be used to cannulate the brachiocephalic vessels and left or right coronary arteries, bypass grafts, and left ventriculography.

2. **Smooth Curved Catheters**
   a. **Cobra:** The tip of the catheter is shaped like the head of a cobra. This is commonly used for renal, visceral, or pelvic angiography or

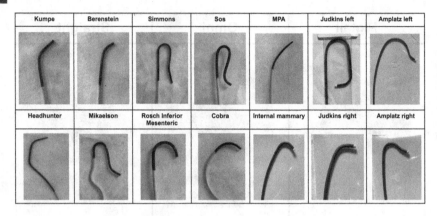

Figure 7.2 Commonly used selective catheters.

crossing the iliac bifurcation. There are three variants, C1, C2, and C3, and each catheter has a progressively widening curve.

b. **Rosch Inferior Mesenteric (RIM):** This is a catheter with a short U-shaped reverse curve. It is good for selecting the inferior mesenteric artery (IMA), and can be useful for selecting the contralateral inferior epigastric artery.

c. **Headhunter:** This catheter has a forward-facing primary curve and is primarily used for head and neck vessels.

3. **Coronary Catheters**

a. **Judkins (Judkins Right [JR] or Judkins Left [JL]):** These catheters come in different configurations depending on if the left or right coronary is to be cannulated. They are commonly used to cannulate native coronary arteries.

b. **Internal Mammary:** Shaped similarly to the JR catheter, but it has a steeply angled tip. It is useful in patients with left internal mammary artery (LIMA) grafts.

c. **Amplatz (Amplatz Right or Amplatz Left):** These catheters also come in different configurations depending on if the left or right coronary is to be cannulated. This is particularly useful if there is nonconventional anatomy. These also come in three variants, with a progressively widening curve.

4. **Complex, Reverse Curved Catheters**

a. **Simmons "Sidewinder":** This is a reverse curve catheter that needs to form either in the aortic arch or over the iliac bifurcation. This catheter is commonly used for the great vessels or visceral angiography. There are three variants, S1, S2, and S3, and each catheter has a progressively widening curve and longer limbs.

b. **Reverse Curve Selective (SOS or Visceral Selective):** This is a reverse curve catheter with a shorter reverse curve than a Simmons Sidewinder. It is commonly used for visceral and renal angiography. These also come in three variants, with a progressively widening curve.

c. **Mikaelson:** It looks similar to a visceral selective catheter, only with a "bump" on the back end to stabilize the catheter within the aorta. It is commonly used for bronchial arteries.

d. **Renal Double Curve (RDC):** This catheter has a downward pointing curve, which is steeper than the cobra catheter. This catheter is designed for renal catheterization.

Microcatheters: These are small catheters that often range from 1.5 to 3Fr in size and are used via a coaxial technique with a larger base catheter. These catheters are very flexible and are optimal for superselective catheterization of small and tortuous vessels and are steered into small vessels using 0.014–0.018 in microwires (2). Microcatheters always need to be longer than their base catheters, and they are often 110–150 cm in length (2).

The measurement of the microcatheters is the same as regular catheters. Therefore, it is important to note that the outer diameter of the microcatheter determines which inner diameter base catheter it fits into (3). In addition, careful consideration must be made about the inner diameter, which can vary to a thousandth of an inch and will determine which embolic devices can be successfully deployed (2). For example, Penumbra Ruby coils require a high-flow microcatheter with an inner diameter of at least 0.025 in and Medtronic Concerto coils are easier to deploy through a standard microcatheter.

There are several microcatheter brands out on the market today. The easiest way to categorize the microcatheters is by function into three categories: standard, high-flow, and anti-reflux or selective occlusion microcatheters.

1. **Standard Microcatheters:** These are end-hole catheters, which are mostly straight tipped, and angled-tipped catheters.

2. **High-Flow Microcatheters:** These catheters are able to be power injected. However, a significant amount of pressure can be transmitted to the vessel, and careful consideration and adjustment of pounds per square inch (psi) must be taken to avoid vessel injury. Commonly used examples are the 2.8Fr Progreat (Terumo) or Renegade Hi-Flo (Boston Scientific).

a. **Renegade Hi-Flo** comes in different variants such as the Fathom, Transend, and STC. These are braided hydrophilic catheters with platinum or steel, which allows for flexibility.

   b. **Progreat (Terumo):** These hydrophilic catheters are made out of Teflon with a Tungsten coil.

3. **Anti-Reflux or Selective Occlusion Microcatheters:** These catheters have either a balloon or anti-reflux cone, which helps prevent non-target embolization. Examples include the Sniper balloon occlusion catheter (Embolx) or Surefire anti-reflux catheters.

Guide Catheters: These are larger catheters commonly ranging from 6 to 8Fr in size. The design is a non-tapered catheter with a stiffer shaft and larger inner diameter, which provide additional support for catheters, wires, coil, balloons, and stents. Guide catheters also come in a variety of different shapes. An important distinction to make is the difference between a guide catheter and an introducer guide, which is essentially a long sheath (3).

Key Points

- Catheter outer diameter is measured in French (1F = 0.33 mm or 3F = 1 mm), inner diameter is measured in inches, and length is measured in centimeters.
- Flow rates for catheters are dependent on the catheter diameter, length, presence of side holes, and pressure rating. These are specified on the packaging. Be careful not to exceed pressure and flow rates to prevent vessel dissection.
- When using selective catheters, rotate at the puncture site and the distal end to gain maximum torque.
- Categorize microcatheters by function into three categories: standard, high-flow, and anti-reflux or selective occlusion microcatheters.
- Diagnostic catheter inner diameter size determines which microcatheter outer diameter can fit for proper coaxial canalization.
- Microcatheters always need to be longer than their base catheters and usually need to be a minimum of 110–150 cm.

References

1. Uberoi R. Interventional Radiology. 1st ed. New York: Oxford University Press; 2009.
2. Kessel D, Robertson I. Interventional Radiology: A Survival Guide. 4th ed. Elsevier; 2016.
3. Rahim S. Pocket Interventional Radiology. 1st ed. Wolters Kluwer; 2018.

CHAPTER 8

CTO TECHNIQUES AND RE-ENTRY DEVICES

John "Will" Perry, Jason Ty Turner, David Hardy

KEYWORDS

chronic total occlusion, re-entry, true lumen, false lumen

LEARNING OBJECTIVES

- Recognize the characteristics of and the challenges that chronic total occlusions (CTOs) present for revascularization
- Understand the basic tools and complementary techniques needed for crossing CTOs
- Develop a basic understanding of how re-entry devices are employed to facilitate difficult true lumen re-entry

Chronic total occlusions (CTOs) are major challenges for revascularization, and are associated with worse post-procedural outcomes compared with stenotic (not fully occluded) lesions. The ability to consistently cross a CTO requires experience and knowledge of the multitude of wires, support catheters, and dedicated CTO re-entry devices that are now available.

Currently, over 40% of patients being treated with peripheral arterial disease and up to 50% of patients with coronary artery disease (CAD) have CTOs. Attempts at recanalization and revascularization should be the only reason to cross CTOs, as the complications involved with crossing can have the potential to convert a relatively stable, chronic ischemia to acute ischemia.

The Lesion

Whether in the coronary or peripheral vascular beds, CTOs generally have similar anatomy and characteristics, several of which can predict the complexity of revascularization. The formation of a long occlusion usually starts with a critical lesion/stenosis from an atherosclerotic plaque that thromboses, forming an adjacent thrombus. This chronic thrombus then propagates thrombus proximally and distally to the culprit lesion/stenosis until the next significant collateral, eventually remodeling to form a fibrous cap. Ischemia-induced angiogenesis then promotes the formation of additional collaterals from existing ones in an attempt by the vasculature to maintain flow to the distal reconstituted segment (Figure 8.1).

The collateralization of CTOs becomes a factor when managing and intervening on occlusions. In the periphery, the proximal and distal CTO caps, length of the lesions (tends to be >50 mm), and involvement of the proximal tibial junctions are elements of complexity that are most challenging for endovascular revascularization.

In coronary CTO crossing, complexity is also a function of lesion morphology. Lesions without a well-defined cap often have neovascular channels running through the plaque into the vasa vasorum of the adventitia. These channels tend to direct a guidewire into the subintimal space. Alternatively, neovascular microchannels that can be found traversing chronic thrombi communicate with the distal true lumen leading to a tapered CTO distal cap. These channels can facilitate the crossing into the distal true lumen if navigated properly.

Imaging

Adequate arteriography is important when considering endovascular recanalization to assess the occlusion length, characteristics, and runoff. Digital subtraction arteriography (DSA) is typically adequate to demonstrate a CTO in the peripheral arteries. In the coronary arteries, DSA is unavailable because of cardiac motion, and the interventionalist relies on the pattern of occlusion and collateral arteries to identify CTOs.

In addition to angiography, intravascular coaxial imaging modalities (e.g., optical coherence tomography [OCT], intravascular ultrasound [IVUS]) can be used to identify lesions, understand CTO morphology, and guide endovascular intervention. These are described more fully in Chapter 13, "Intravascular Imaging Modalities (OCT and IVUS)."

Tools for Crossing

The use of specific CTO wires and support catheters has led to increasing success with recanalization of CTOs. Most CTOs are crossed in the subintimal plane using a hydrophilic guidewire and hydrophilic support catheter. When determining the wire for crossing, the key attributes to consider are tip stiffness, torque response, rail support, and lubricity. Tip stiffness impacts crossability, especially for heavily calcified lesions that require significant pressure to penetrate caps and support continued lesion dissection. Torque response refers to the ability of the guidewire to navigate and select side branches. Rail support is a function of the guidewire stiffness and can enhance pushability and device support. The lubricity of the wire may decrease friction forces and enhance crossability but decreases tactile feedback. A hydrophilic coated wire has an increased lubricity for decreased frictional forces. The size of the wire will depend on the intervening segment, most commonly being 0.035", 0.018", or 0.014" wires (but can drop to sizes of 0.009–0.010" with specialty coronary wires) (see Table 8.1).

For added support and pushability, dedicated support catheters are frequently used to cross. These catheters are gradually and intermittently advanced over the guidewires to push across occlusions. The combination of hydrophilic guidewire and catheter with a stiff tip can be very effective in crossing. Table 8.2 lists the commonly used support catheters and sizes for crossing.

Techniques of Crossing

There are several different strategies to crossing CTOs. Regardless of the approach, choose the access site with the shortest distance to the CTO, antegrade or retrograde. At times, a dual antegrade and retrograde approach to crossing an occlusion can be required.

Table 8.1 Wires Typically Used for Crossing

	Hydrophilic Coating	CTO
Boston Scientific	0.014": Journey™, V-14™ 0.018": V-18™	Victory™ 0.014 and 0.018"
Abbott	0.014": HT Command™, Pilot™ 0.018": HT Connect	0.018": HT Connect Flex, HT Connect
Terumo	Glidewire® 0.018" and 0.014"	—
Asahi	—	0.014": Miraclebros™, Confianza™ 0.018": Astato™
Asahi (Coronary)	0.009": Fielder XT 0.010": Gaia 1	0.014": Miracle 3, 4.5, 6 0.014": Ultimate Bros 3

Table 8.2 Dedicated Support Catheters (in inches)

Boston Scientific	Spectranetics	Bard	Vascular Solutions	Covidien	Cook	Terumo
Rubicon™	Quick-Cross™	Seeker™	Minnie™	Trailblazer™	CXI™	NaviCross™
0.014	0.014	0.014	0.014	0.014	—	—
0.018	0.018	0.018	0.018	0.018	0.018	—
0.035	0.035	0.035	0.035	0.035	0.035	0.035

- **Intraluminal Crossing:** The intraluminal approach requires no re-entry and provides the shortest possible reconstruction. Position the sheath close to the CTO to give added support and pushability. Typically, either straight-tipped or angled hydrophilic guidewires are used to probe the occlusion initially. Use a smaller platform when working with smaller vessels. To gain additional support a dedicated support/crossing catheter is used over the guidewire; having a platform with adequate support and pushability is paramount to the success of crossing. Probe, drill, and push the guidewire into the occlusion until advancement stops. The catheter is then passed over the guidewire, and the guidewire is advanced while rotating the tip to bore into the occlusion. The catheter is advanced gradually and intermittently over the guidewire as advancements are made. The guidewire should always be a few millimeters out from the tip of the catheters. These rotating and drilling maneuvers of the guidewire help establish an intraluminal crossing path. The steps are used incrementally until the CTO is crossed (Figure 8.2a–c). Occasionally, the guidewire is removed and contrast can be flushed into catheter to determine the progress and position. To stay intraluminal, avoid forming loops in the guidewire, as this may be a sign that the wire has passed in the subintimal plane. There are specialized catheters designed to drill through CTOs without a leading wire, and these are available commercially.
- **Soft Plaque/Loose Tissue Tracking/Acute Myocardial (MI) Cases:** These are usually performed with an intermediate-strength hydrophilic wire with ~1 gram tip that is shaped with a 45–60-degree angle several millimeters from the end to allow for storability. These soft lesions are often crossed smoothly with minimal twirling. If difficulty arises penetrating the distal cap a microcatheter can be advanced over the wire to allow for greater pushability or exchange of wire for a stiffer tapered tip.
- **Subintimal Crossing:** The subintimal approach utilizes a potential space between the layers of the vessel wall where a wire and catheter may pass and then "re-enters" the true lumen of the vessel. This re-entry may occur spontaneously or with the assistance of a special re-entry device. When

the CTO is crossed subintimally, an attempt is made to re-enter the true lumen distal to the occlusion close to the reconstituting collaterals. These collaterals identify the point of where re-entry is more easily achieved. The technique of subintimal approach is similar in many ways to the intraluminal approach described above. The wire is probed, drilled, and pushed into the stump of the occluded artery, usually at the arterial wall and plaque interface that is opposite a large collateral. The tip of the guidewire will engage the plaque and form a loop at the flexible portion of the wire. The loop is advanced a few centimeters, and the support catheter is then advanced intermittently to the base of the loop without straightening the wire. The loop is then further advanced along the subintimal plane down the occlusion, and this sequence of wire and catheter advancement occurs in a stepwise fashion down the occlusion. Take care to watch the trajectory of the wire to ensure that is it coursing along the anticipated pathway of the artery. In the periphery, continued use of road-mapping can allow for quick assessment of the distance from the guidewire to the termination of the occlusion. Contrast administration via the sheath or support catheter will identify the reconstituting collateral during crossing. The guidewire loop and catheter should be pushed to the area of reconstitution and usually the loop will re-enter the true lumen at this point with a change in the wire formation (Figure 8.3a–c). If there is difficulty re-entering at the point of reconstitution, an angled tip support catheter can be angled toward the true lumen and the wire can be directed toward the true lumen. Another option is to balloon angioplasty the plaque to fracture and create a re-entry space. To confirm re-entry the catheter is advanced, guidewire is removed, and contrast administered to obtain a distal lumenogram; IVUS may also be used to identify wire presence within the true lumen.

For percutaneous coronary intervention (PCI), subintimal crossing is less preferred than remaining within the true lumen but is an accepted and invaluable technique. The wire is completely within the false lumen when it bends back on itself and advances with the base of the J-portion of wire freely with little resistance. Re-entry into the distal true lumen remains the crux of this technique and is the leading cause of crossing failure and increased risk of myocardial infarction.

Difficulty with Re-Entry

If re-entry is not successful by changing support catheters, balloon angioplasty, or with exchanges of wires, a dedicated re-entry device can be used to facilitate entering the true lumen (Table 8.3). These devices typically require gentle

Table 8.3 Re-Entry Devices

Device Name	Manufacturer	Coronary/ Peripheral	Guidewire Compatibility (inches)	Method of Re-Entry
Outback™	Cordis	Peripheral	0.014	Radiopaque markers utilized to orient a port through which curved hypodermic re-entry needle is deployed to puncture intimal flap and allow guidewire advancement into the true lumen
Pioneer Plus™	Philips	Peripheral	0.014	IVUS-assisted orientation of a port for deployment of a hypodermic re-entry needle to puncture the intimal flap and allow advancement of a guidewire into the true lumen
Enteer™	Medtronic	Peripheral	0.014; 0.018	Flat balloon is utilized to self-orient device within the subintimal space and direct a port for deployment of a hypodermic re-entry needle to puncture the intimal flap and allow advancement of a guidewire into the true lumen
OffRoad™	Boston Scientific	Peripheral	0.014	Conical balloon is utilized to tent the intimal flap over the end of the catheter, thereby directing the catheter end toward the intraluminal space. A needle cannula is then advanced to puncture the intimal flap and allow guidewire advancement into the true lumen
Stingray™ (±CrossBoss™)	Boston Scientific	Coronary	0.014; 0.018	Flat balloon is utilized to orient the device in the subintimal space, which has multiple angled re-entry ports through which the intimal flap can be probed with a guidewire to identify an optimal site for puncture and re-entry. Often used in conjunction with the CrossBoss™ catheter, a blunt, atraumatic support catheter designed for intraluminal or subintimal crossing

dilation of the subintimal tract via small caliber angioplasty with 3- or 4-mm balloons or passage of a guiding catheter. A 0.014″ support wire is used for the devices and the device must be passed to the end of the guidewire, which does not provide a sturdy system over which the device will work. Typically, the guidewire and catheter are advanced past the occlusion in the subintimal plane. The guidewire is exchanged for a 0.014″ guidewire and the wire is advanced past the occlusion in the subintimal space. The support catheter is removed and the device is then loaded onto the guidewire. These devices are discussed in more detail below, but most use a re-entry cannula or needle that is directed toward the true lumen by use of markers. The needle or cannula is then placed intro the true lumen though the subintimal space, and a 0.014″ or 0.018″ guidewire is then advanced into the true lumen distally (Figure 8.4).

Despite the advances and techniques described attempts at crossing may still be unsuccessful, even in the most experienced of hands. In order to reliably and consistently cross CTOs, the operator must have a vast understanding and experience with the wires, support catheters, devices, and access techniques. The complexity of CTOs and the progression of these advanced atherosclerotic disease states pose a continuing challenge for these patients and operators.

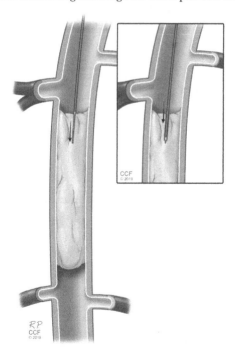

Figure 8.1 Picture of CTO with collaterals and thrombus. (Abbreviation: *CTO*, chronic total occlusions.)

Key Points

- Chronic thrombus forms proximal and distal to a hemodynamically significant stenosis with the formation of collateralization, which becomes important factors during interventions.
- There are a multitude of wires and catheters used for crossing lesions, the most frequently used setup includes hydrophilic wire with a dedicated support catheter to allow for added support and pushability while the wire and catheter are advanced in a stepwise fashion.
- The techniques for crossing an occlusion include intraluminal and subintimal. Subintimal, which is the most common, requires entering the occlusion in the "subintimal" plane while advancing the wire until it re-enters within the true lumen distal to the occlusion.
- In difficult cases where re-entry into the true lumen cannot be achieved with wire skills, dedicated re-entry devices are available to help with re-establishing the true lumen.

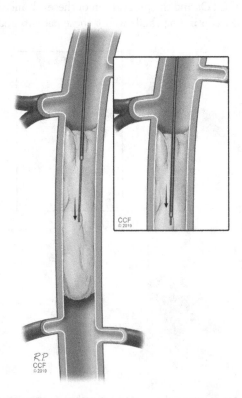

Figure 8.2 (A) Intraluminal crossing.

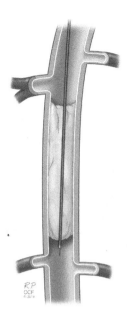

Figure 8.2 (B)

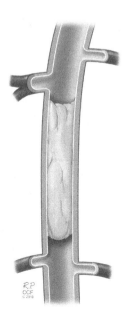

Figure 8.2 (C)

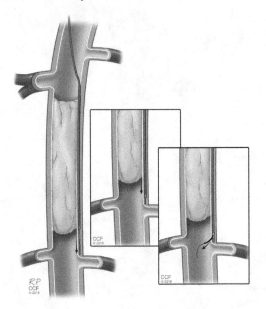

Figure 8.3 (A) Subintimal crossing.

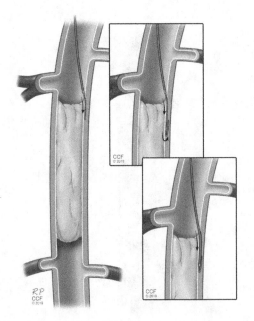

Figure 8.3 (B)

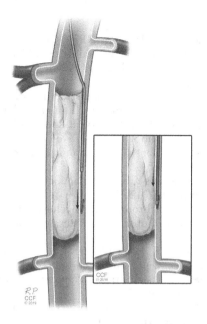

Figure 8.3 (C)

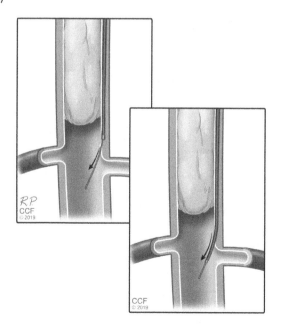

Figure 8.4 Re-entry technique.

References

1. Hirsch AT, Haskal ZJ, Hertzer NR. ACC/AHA Guidelines for the Management of Patients with Peripheral Arterial Disease (Lower Extremity, Renal, Mesenteric, and Abdominal Aortic). Jur Vasc Interv Radiol. 2006;47(6):1239–7312.
2. Bargellini I, Scatena A, Cioni R, Cicorelli A. Primary infrainguinal subintimal angioplasty in diabetic patients primary infrainguinal subintimal angioplasty in diabetic patients. Cardiovasc Intervent Radiol. 2008;31(4):713–722.
3. Ramjas G, Thurley P, Habib S. The use of a re-entry catheter in recanalization of chronic inflow occlusions of the common iliac artery. Cardiovasc Interv Ther. 2008;31(3):650–654.
4. Owens CD, Yeghiarazians Y, editors. Handbook of Endovascular Peripheral Interventions. Springer; 2012.
5. Tajti P, Brilakis ES. Chronic total occlusion percutaneous coronary intervention: evidence of controversies. J Am Heart Assoc. 2018; 7(e006732):1–14.
6. Karacsonyi J, Alaswad K, Jaffer FA, Yeh RW, Patel M, Bahadorani J, et al. Use of intravascular imaging during chronic total occlusion percutaneous coronary intervention: insights from a contemporary multicenter registry. J Am Heart Assoc. 2016;5(8):1–13.
7. Schneider PA. Guidewire-catheter skills. In: Endovascular Skills. 3rd ed. London: Healthcare Informa; 2009; p. 57–61.

CHAPTER 9

ANGIOPLASTY BALLOONS AND TECHNIQUE

Ann H. Kim, Norman H. Kumins

KEYWORDS

angioplasty, insufflator, balloon, cutting balloon, drug-coated

LEARNING OBJECTIVES

- Understand the mechanism of balloon angioplasty and vessel remodeling
- Describe the structural parameters of balloon catheters
- Explain the indications, limitations, and complications of balloon angioplasty
- List available options in selecting a balloon for a specific use

Introduction

Transluminal balloon angioplasty is a procedure used to improve blood flow by increasing the diameter of a narrowed or diseased artery or vein. Arterial dilation by the passage of a series of sequentially larger dilators was first described by Dotter and Judkins in the mid-1960s (1). Arterial dilation with the use of a balloon catheter was first described by Gruntzig and Hopff for treatment of an atherosclerotic plaque in a coronary artery (2).

Angioplasty is performed using a catheter with a balloon mounted on the end of the shaft. The balloon is inflated inside a vessel within the stenotic region, thereby, dilating the specific lesion. When performed in an atherosclerotic arterial plaque, it causes a controlled longitudinal fracture within the plaque-lined intima, separating it from the media and adventitia. The arterial lumen increases by flattening the plaque and stretching the media and adventitia. This yields a controlled dissection which then initiates a remodeling process, starting with platelet deposition and ending with re-endothelialization (3).

Balloon Design

The balloon device is created by wrapping the balloon around the shaft of a dual-lumen delivery catheter (Figure 9.1). One lumen is for passage over a guidewire and the other lumen is connected to the balloon to allow for its inflation. Most often the balloon is inflated with an inflation device, which indicates the pressure applied to the balloon. Typically, there are one or

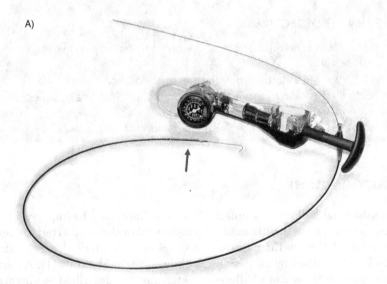

A)

Figure 9.1 Typical peripheral balloon. (A) Balloon, guidewire, and attached inflation device. Note that the balloon is mounted to the distal end of the balloon catheter (arrow) and the inflation device is attached to the opposite end.

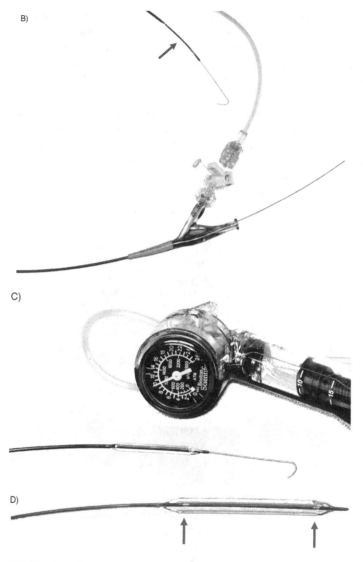

Figure 9.1 (*Continued*)
(B) Balloon in the uninflated state. Note the balloon wrapped around one end of the catheter (arrow) and the two lumens at the opposite end. The wire can be seen exiting from one lumen and the other is connected to a balloon inflation device. (C) Balloon in the inflated state. The pressure applied to the balloon can be seen on the inflation device. This balloon is inflated to 10 atm. (D) Close-up view of an inflated angioplasty balloon. Note the balloon is marked with two radiopaque markers (arrows) that indicate the end of the area being treated. The remainder of the balloon tapers as the balloon "shoulder," which would not be in contact with the vessel wall

more radiopaque markers that indicate the location of the balloon on the catheter, so it can be appropriately positioned under fluoroscopic imaging. Short coronary balloons typically have a single marker in the center of the balloon, peripheral balloons typically have markers on each balloon end, and very long balloons often have markers on each end and another in the middle (Figure 9.2).

The angioplasty balloon has multiple structural parameters. Balloons come in different sizes that correspond to the balloon diameter, balloon length, and length of the balloon catheter. Diameters start as small as 1.0 mm and can go beyond 40 mm (specialty aortic balloons). Smaller balloons typically increase by 0.5-mm increments until they reach a diameter of 5 mm, then increase by 1 mm up until 10 mm, and then increase by 2 mm up to about 24 mm. Balloon

A)

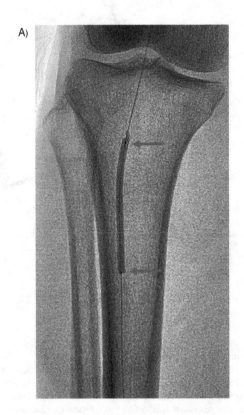

Figure 9.2 View under fluoroscopy of various balloons in the inflated state. The balloon is inflated with dilute iodinated contrast medium allowing the lumen to appear under X-ray visualization. (A) Short peripheral balloon. Note the radiopaque markers indicating the outer edge of the balloon (arrows).

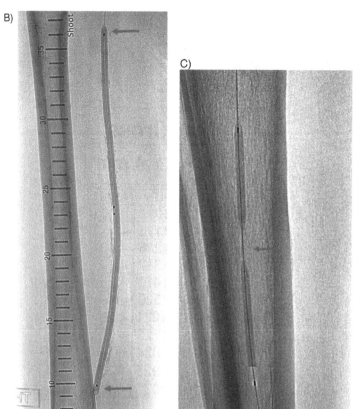

Figure 9.2 (*Continued*)
(B) Long peripheral balloon. There are radiopaque markers on both ends (arrows) and a double marker to indicate the center of the balloon. (C) Balloon partially inflated. Note the waist in the middle of the balloon at the location of the arterial stenosis (arrow).

length describes the length of the balloon segment and range from about 10 mm to greater than 300 mm. The catheter itself that delivers the balloon can be as short as 40 cm or longer than 170 cm. Selection of the catheter length depends on the site of the lesion to be treated and the access point. If access is in the groin and the lesion is in the ipsilateral iliac artery, then a short catheter will reach. If the target, however, is distal on the contralateral limb, then a long catheter length will be needed.

Another key feature is balloon compliance, which is defined by the level of elasticity or deformability at a given applied force. Balloons can be created from a variety of materials, each of which respond differently to pressure. Balloons can be compliant, allowing them to deform in direct relation to

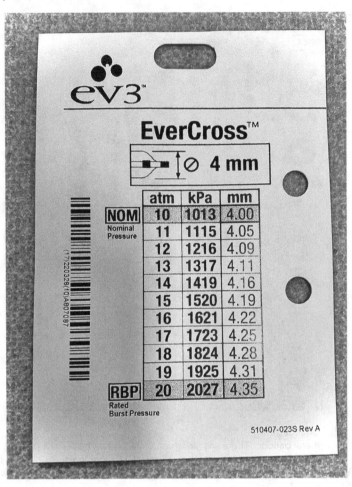

Figure 9.3 Typical compliance chart for a semi-compliant peripheral balloon.

the pressure applied or be non-compliant where the balloon stays the same size irrespective of the pressure applied. Most peripheral balloons are semi-compliant and are typically packaged with a chart that lists the expected size of the balloon at a given pressure (Figure 9.3). The nominal pressure describes the pressure at which the balloon reaches its indicated size, and the rated burst pressure describes the pressure at which the balloon is expected to fracture. A balloon with low compliance allows for adequate force to be applied to the lesion without significant overdistension of uninvolved vessel. Compliant balloons should be used cautiously because the balloon can be expanded beyond the vessel diameter and lead to rupture.

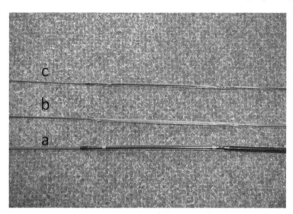

Figure 9.4 Various balloon catheters ordered by size of wire and wire configuration. These are all 4-mm diameter balloons. Note how the balloon profile decreases as the wire size decreases. (a) A 0.035″ balloon mounted on a 0.035 wire. (b) A 0.018″ balloon mounted on a 0.018 wire. (c) A 0.014″ balloon mounted on a 0.014 wire. As the wire sizes decrease so do the balloon catheter profiles.

The balloon catheter is delivered to the target lesion over a guidewire. The balloon catheter itself is sized based on the wire diameter over which it will pass. The smaller the wire, the smaller the crossing profile of the balloon catheter. Balloon catheters typically are sized by passing over standard wire sizes of 0.014″, 0.018″, and 0.035″ (Figure 9.4). Balloons can be "over the wire," which means that the entire catheter passes over the guidewire. They also come as "rapid exchange" or "monorail," which means that the wire passes out of the catheter close to the proximal end allowing the balloon and wire to be controlled by a single operator and the balloon to be more quickly loaded and removed.

Some balloons are designed to cut or score the lesion. Cutting balloons have small, longitudinally mounted blades protruding from the balloon that score or cut into the lesion when the balloon is inflated (Figure 9.5). This technique is useful to treat stiff or calcified plaque allowing for improved vessel expansion. Scoring balloons are similarly designed but have wires mounted to the outside of the balloon instead of blades. They work in a similar fashion but make a less aggressive cut on the lesion.

Angioplasty Technique

When balloon angioplasty is indicated the first step in treatment is to obtain secure access proximal to the lesion with a sheath. The sheath allows for the introduction and removal of interventional devices and provides a mechanism

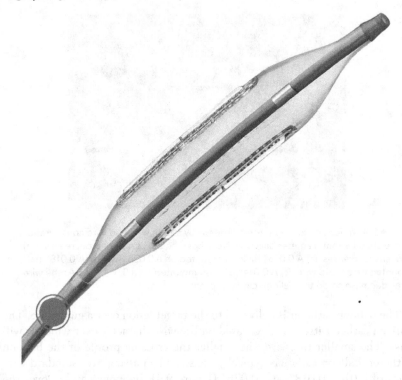

Figure 9.5 Cutting the balloon in the inflated state. Note the blades oriented longitudinally on the balloon.

to perform angiography pre- and post-treatment. The sheath should be placed at a reasonable distance from the intended treatment site. Prior to crossing the stenosis, the patient is typically systemically anticoagulated.

The next step is to cross the lesion with a guidewire (Figure 9.6). There are various techniques and wire and catheter combinations to use depending on the nature and location of the lesion. Once across the area of concern, the operator selects the most appropriate wire and balloon to treat the diseased segment, taking into account wire size, balloon diameter, balloon length, shaft length, and balloon compliance. Estimation of vessel diameter can be made by measuring the vessel immediately proximal or distal to the stenosis.

The lesion must be mapped out appropriately to allow the balloon to be appropriately placed under fluoroscopy. The operator can use bony landmarks, a ruler, contrast injection through the sheath, or road-mapping to accomplish placement. The balloon is inflated using a dilute mixture of contrast and saline such that the outline of the balloon can be seen fluoroscopically. The balloon is left inflated for a predetermined period of time. It is then deflated and removed. A post-angioplasty angiographic image is then obtained.

Balloon inflation is typically accomplished with the use of an insufflation device. The device has a chamber that can be filled with diluted contrast medium. This chamber is connected via a Luer lock to the inflation port on the balloon. There is a threaded plunger mounted on the chamber that pushes the contrast mixture under pressure into the balloon when turned in a clockwise direction. A pressure gauge is connected to the chamber so the pressure applied to the balloon is known.

When treating a high-grade arterial stenosis, sequential dilation is often desirable. A balloon with a smaller diameter is inflated within the lesion prior to the appropriate sized balloon. This gradual dilation decreases the risk for arterial dissection and arterial perforation.

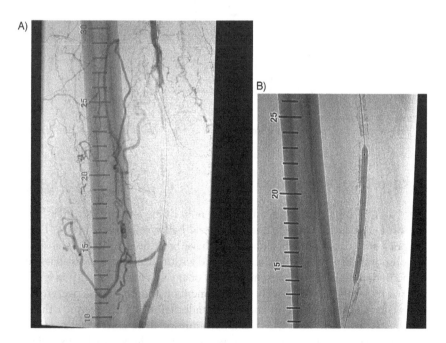

Figure 9.6 Typical angioplasty technique. (A) Angiographic image of the arterial occlusion in the SFA with a wire across the lesion. Note the radiopaque tape marking the length and location of the occlusion. (B) Balloon inflated across the occlusion. (Abbreviation: *SFA*, superficial femoral artery.)

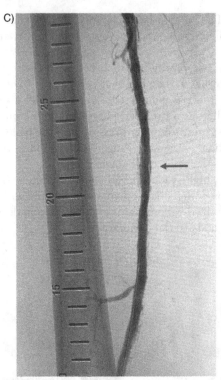

Figure 9.6 (*Continued*)
(C) Post-angioplasty result. Note a small amount of non–flow-limiting dissection (arrow).

Drug-Coated Balloons

One of the most exciting advances in balloon angioplasty has been the development of drug-coated peripheral balloons (DCBs) (4–6). These balloons are coated with paclitaxel and have been used to treat stenoses in femoropopliteal arteries, tibial arteries, and within arteriovenous fistulas used for hemodialysis access. The Achilles' heel of any vascular intervention is neo-intimal hyperplasia, which is the development of smooth muscle overgrowth incited by the denudation of the vessel endothelium. This overgrowth can be arrested by paclitaxel, which is an antimitotic drug used to treat cancer. Paclitaxel-coated peripheral balloons have been shown to be especially beneficial in treating femoropopliteal arterial atherosclerotic disease and have shown promise in treating arteriovenous fistulas and grafts. Current studies using DCBs in tibial arteries are ongoing.

Results/Complications

The ideal lesion for angioplasty is a short focal stenosis. The longer the lesion length, more of the vessel is at risk for restenosis. Controlled arterial dissection is an intended consequence of angioplasty; it is how the balloon dilates the vessel. This dissection, however, can be uncontrolled and severe enough to be flow limiting (Figure 9.7). Untreated, these dissections can cause arterial thrombosis. Additionally, angioplasty-treated lesions often recoil, especially if they are heavily calcified. Balloon angioplasty, therefore, is often not adequate stand-alone therapy and must be combined with other modalities such as atherectomy or stent placement. If the lesion is especially dense, calcified or bulky angioplasty can lead to arterial perforation. The operator must keep the possibility of perforation in mind, and techniques to treat this complication should be considered before intervention occurs.

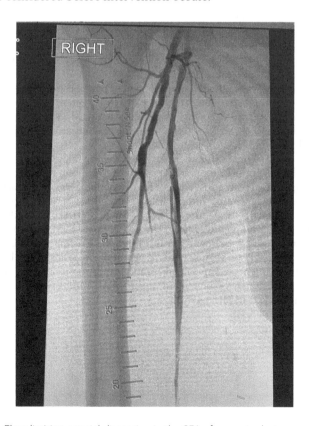

Figure 9.7 Flow-limiting arterial dissection in the SFA after angioplasty. (Abbreviation: *SFA*, superficial femoral artery.)

83

Key Points

- Balloon angioplasty is a basic technique used to expand the lumen of an artery or vein. It works by inflating a balloon wrapped around the shaft of a catheter that is positioned over a guidewire.
- There are numerous structural parameters that define the characteristics of the balloon. These characteristics allow for different uses in different clinical situations.
- Complications of balloon angioplasty include arterial recoil, dissection, and perforation. The operator must be prepared to treat these complications if they arise.
- Paclitaxel-coated balloons have been shown to improve patency when used in the femoropopliteal segment. Additional studies are ongoing assessing their uses on other locations.

References

1. Dotter CT, Judkins MP. Transluminal treatment of arteriosclerotic obstruction: description of a new technic and a preliminary report of its application. Circulation. 1964;30:654–670.
2. Gruntzig A, Kumpe DA. Technique of percutaneous transluminal angioplasty with the Gruntzig balloon catheter. Am J Roentgenol. 1979;132:547–552.
3. Castaneda-Zuniga W, Formanek A, Tadavarthy M, Vlodaver Z, Edwards J, Zollikofer C, et al. The mechanism of balloon angioplasty. Radiology. 1980;135:565–571.
4. Scheinert D, Duda S, Zeller T, Krankenberg H, Ricke J, Bosiers M, et al. The Levant I (Lutonix paclitaxel-coated balloon for the prevention of femoropopliteal restenosis) trial for femoropopliteal revascularization. J Am Coll Cardiol Cardiovasc Interv. 2014;7(1):10–19.
5. Rosenfield K, Jaff MR, White CJ, Rocha-Singh K. Trial of a paclitaxel-coated balloon for femoropopliteal artery disease. N Engl J Med. 2015;373:145–153.
6. Gunnar T, Laird J, Schneider P, Brodman M, Krishnan P, Micari A, et al. Drug-coated balloon versus standard percutaneous transluminal angioplasty for the treatment of superficial femoral and popliteal peripheral artery disease: 12-month results from the IN.PACT SFA Randomized Trial. Circulation. 2014;131(5):495–502.

CHAPTER 10

STENTS

Ravi N. Ambani, Jae S. Cho

LEARNING OBJECTIVES

- Understand the indications, contraindications, and complications associated with stenting
- Understand different types of stents
- Understand basic techniques required in stent placement

Introduction

Currently, various endovascular therapies exist for the treatment of peripheral arterial disease (PAD), including balloon angioplasty, drug-coated balloon angioplasty, bare metal stents (BMS), drug-eluting stents, and atherectomy. These technologies work in different ways, some displace plaque by shear force while others attempt to remove the plaque burden directly. Intravascular stents provide an internal scaffolding across a stenotic or occluded blood vessel to maintain patency and re-establish flow (1). Although balloon angioplasty was widely practiced for more than 15 years, the introduction of stent technology broadened the scope of endovascular therapy in multiple ways: (1) treatment of complications of balloon angioplasty, (2) occlusion or long lesions that would have required open reconstructive surgery, (3) treatment of high-risk patients who would have been denied an open surgical therapy, and (4) treatment of aneurysm with stent grafts (2).

Arterial stenting follows the same principles and indications that have been established for open intervention. In the lower extremities, disabling claudication and critical limb ischemia are the main indications for treatment. Similarly, patients who present with severe arm claudication and ischemic

Table 10.1 Indications for Peripheral Stent Placement

Lower Extremity:

- Severe, disabling claudication
- Lifestyle-limiting claudication refractory to lifestyle modification and exercise regimen
- Ischemic rest pain
- Ischemic non-healing ulcers

Upper Extremity:

- Severe arm claudication with subclavian stenosis
- Subclavian steal syndrome
- Ischemic ulcers

Visceral:

- Medically refractory hypertension on three or more medications with evidence of renal artery stenosis
- Mesenteric ischemia with evidence of celiac artery and/or superior mesenteric artery stenosis

Carotid:

- Carotid stenosis with high operative risk including restenosis after previous endarterectomy, radiation to the neck, and high anatomic lesions

---

ulcers of the hand may benefit from endovascular stenting. Visceral stenting focuses on the treatment of patients with medically refractory hypertension due to renal artery stenosis and mesenteric ischemia from celiac artery and superior mesenteric artery stenosis. Carotid stenting is reserved for patients who are high operative risk for conventional carotid endarterectomy. The indications for peripheral vascular stent placement are summarized in Table 10.1.

When stent placement is planned ahead of time and performed without first performing balloon angioplasty, it is called primary stenting. This works best in situations with recurrent stenosis, occlusion, orificial lesions of aortic branch vessels, and embolizing lesions. Primary stenting is performed usually for renal, carotid, and aortoiliac lesions. It assumes higher cost and procedural risk. Selective stent placement is performed when the cost and risk of stent placement is not justified. It is performed when the results of balloon angioplasty are not satisfactory (i.e., residual stenosis > 30%), persistent pressure gradient, flow-limiting dissection, or perforation. Heavily calcified lesions or lesions with high risk for distal embolism would be best served with a covered stent. When anatomically feasible, aneurysms can be treated with covered stent grafts. Indications for stent placement have expanded steadily since its introduction. As new advances in stenting technologies are developed and introduced, the areas of treatment with stents will continue to broaden.

In general, there are few contraindications to stenting. In rare cases, patients may be allergic to the metal components of the stent, most often nitinol. In any location, a total occlusion in a patient who is good surgical risk should be considered for bypass as there is strong evidence in support of vein bypass and patency. Relative limitations may exist in patients with pre-existing renal insufficiency due to need for contrast during these procedures and in pregnancy as radiation is contraindicated.

Complications of stenting are uncommon but are similar to those of angiography and angioplasty. Any endovascular intervention is associated with the risk of infection, bleeding, arterial trauma, and distal embolism. Carotid artery stenting and any aortic arch catheterization and manipulation can lead to stroke. A rare complication with angioplasty and stenting is acute vessel occlusion, which is often due to dissection and/or plaque shift at the end of the stent and requires immediate treatment with thrombolytic therapy, open surgery, or even emergency bypass (3).

Stent Types

Stents by design can be differentiated based on their composition material, design, and deployment system. In this section, we will address the mechanical properties of the stents followed by the variable deployment systems and in which location of the body these are indicated.

Current stent technology is based on metallic composition. The different composites include stainless steel, nickel-titanium (nitinol), and cobalt-chromium. Physical properties of these metals are summarized in Table 10.2. In general, stents can come as BMSs (Figure 10.1a,b) or covered with a fabric (e.g., polytetrafluoroethylene [PTFE] as a covered stent [Figure 10.1c]). The three main properties in the construction of stents are elastic modulus, yield

Table 10.2 Physical Properties of Stent Materials

Property	Stainless Steel	Cobalt-Chromium	Nitinol	Titanium
Elastic modulus	High	Very high	Very low	Low
Strength	Medium	High	High	High
Stiffness	Very high	High	Very low	Moderate
Radiodensity	Low	Moderate	Low	Moderate
MRI compatible	No	Yes	Yes	Yes

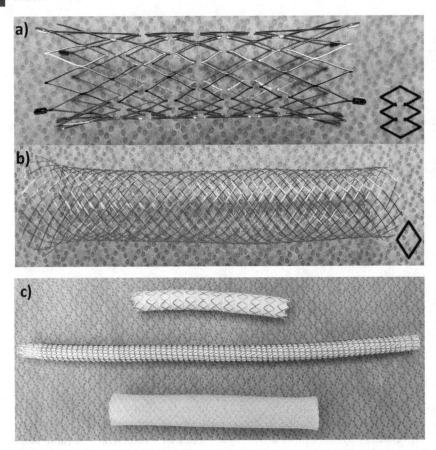

Figure 10.1 Examples of basic types of stent construction. (a) Bare metal stent (open cell). (b) Bare metal stent (closed cell). (c) Covered stent (three different examples displayed).

strength, and tensile strength. Elastic modulus is defined as the ratio of stress to strain in the elastic range of deformation. It measures an object's resistance to being deformed elastically upon application of a stress. Yield strength is the ability of a metal to resist deformation; metals with a high yield strength will maintain their original conformation unless subjected to a force that exceeds it, leading to permanent deformation. Finally, tensile strength relates to the ability to withstand longitudinal force prior to fracturing (4).

Stainless steel was used in the first generation of bare metal stents and was characterized by good radial strength and prevention of recoil, but due to the thicker struts there was an association with restenosis. Due to the predominance of iron in the metal, it is not very radio-opaque and is not magnetic resonance imaging compatible. Cobalt alloy has higher elastic modulus, yield strength, and density at a smaller profile than stainless steel. Thus, it has equal radial strength and better radio-opacity and restenosis rates. **Nitinol**, comprised of 55% **ni**ckel and 45% **ti**tanium, is characterized by very low elastic modulus and high yield and tensile strength making it an ideal alloy for stent construction. One specific aspect of nitinol stents is their transformation temperature. Largely set to 30°C, these stents can be constrained and manipulated into a delivery system at any temperature below this. Once deployed and rewarmed by the native tissues, it resumes predetermined size and form (4).

The next aspect of stent creation and design is scaffold structure (5). Stents are classified into two main categories: tube and modular. Regarding tube stent construction, coil stents are formed from coiling of a wire into a circular stack forming the scaffolding. In contrast, slotted tube stents are created by using a metallic tube and then laser etching the intended stent design. Coil tube stents are characterized by goof flexibility but poor radial forces and have been associated with a high rate of restenosis. Slotted tube stents exhibit more radial force but are less flexible and harder to deploy than the coiled tube stents. Modular stents have replaced both tube stents due to their construction design which was aimed to combat the limitations of the prior stents. Modular stents are designed using repeated modules that are then fused together to construct a tube, a design which increased its flexibility and side branch accessibility. Modular stents are either designed with open or closed cells.

Open cell stents have cells that are not connected on all sides, while closed cell stents have cells which are connected on all sides. Closed cell design reduces the prolapsing of plaque through the stent and has increased radial force. On the other hand, open cell design allows for more flexibility and branch accessibility and is able to conform better to tortuous anatomy. Currently in the market, modular, open cell designed stents predominate.

Another aspect of stent design is drug elution technology. Drugs that retard intimal hyperplasia (resulting in restenosis and occlusion) are impregnated onto a bare metal stent backbone using a polymer. While there are a variety of drugs available for elution, the predominant drug used in peripheral stents at present is paclitaxel. Drug-eluting stents were developed to reduce the high rate of in-stent restenosis and need for further revascularization procedures. Drug elution is available for both stents and balloons. It is primarily indicated for recurrent stenosis at present (6).

While multiple aforementioned features can be used to describe and categorize a stent, from a practical standpoint, there are two type of stents:

Table 10.3 Balloon-Expandable and Self-Expanding Stents

Attribute	Balloon-Expandable	Self-Expanding
Appearance	Partial Deployment/Inflation Full Deployment/Inflation	Partial Deployment Full Deployment
Delivery system	Balloon-mounted	Constrained on catheter
Size at delivery	Nominal diameter after balloon inflation	Nominal diameter with expansion at body temperature
Post-dilation required	No	Yes, for opposition to vessel wall
Ability to size > nominal	Yes (i.e., VBX and Palmaz)	No
Material	Stainless steel or cobalt-chromium alloy	Nitinol
Use	Focal, calcified lesions requiring high precision (i.e., renals)	Longer lesions subject to movement (i.e., superficial femoral)
Precision	Superior	Inferior
Anatomic constraints	Susceptible to external compression and rotational forces (i.e., neck and extremities)	Resistant to external compression and rotational forces

Balloon Expandable Stents (BES) and Self-Expanding Stents (SES). The main differences between BES and SES are detailed in Table 10.3. BES are, in general, rigid and do not conform to any tortuosity or any change in vessel diameter subject to crimping by external forces. As such they are best suited for short, focal lesions (i.e., aortic branch vessels) and avoided in areas of flexion (i.e., popliteal arteries) or areas prone to external compression (i.e., carotid arteries). Commercially available BES have a metal scaffold and are pre-mounted onto a balloon, between 2 radiopaque markers, that are slightly longer than the stent length. The BES stent is designed to be expanded to a certain size known as the nominal diameter and length. An insufflator (as described in Chapter, "Angioplasty Balloons and Technique") must be used to deploy a BES to expand the stent to its nominal size. When an operator is mounting a stent onto a balloon, the same length balloon or longer balloon should be chosen. The stent should be mounted such that the end of the stent is flush with either the proximal or distal radiopaque marker. The stent is secured in position by circumferentially crimping the stent on the balloon with fingers such that the stent should not slide on the balloon.

SES, on the other hand, are relatively more flexible, resistant to external compression and available in longer lengths. They are created at a set diameter and then constrained to a smaller size in a delivery catheter for implantation. When the constraining element is removed, the stent expands to its preformed size. However, they are less accurate and are more prone to movement and may foreshorten during deployment. They are better suited for longer lesions and mobile regions of the body. In most cases, balloon angioplasty is then performed to ensure the stent is well-opposed to the treated vessel.

Stenting Technique

When stenting is necessary, size selection and delivery are of paramount importance. Undersizing a stent may result in migration while oversizing may rupture or tear the vessel. After obtaining a digitally subtracted image, bony landmarks or a radiopaque ruler may be utilized to determine the diameter and length of a stent. The inflated balloon profile may also serve as a guide to sizing the stent or intravascular ultrasound may be used for exact measurements.

For optimal delivery and deployment of a BES, the appropriate sheath and dilator combination is passed through the lesion. The dilator is then removed, and the sheath is flushed. The BES is placed through the valve of the sheath and positioned in the desired location while still sheathed. The location of the stent on the balloon is verified before the sheath is withdrawn. If the stent has moved on the balloon, the balloon and the stent should be removed and reloaded. Once the location of the stent is noted to be satisfactory both on the balloon and across the lesion, the sheath is withdrawn, exposing both the stent and the balloon. The stent is deployed under fluoroscopic guidance by inflation of the balloon.

On the other hand, unlike for BES, the sheath and dilator do not need to be passed through the lesion before the stent is brought into position for SES. SES should be oversized by 1–2 mm so that they exert continuous outward force at the site of treatment. The stents have a fixed diameter and cannot be over-dilated beyond their nominal size. Prior to stenting, the lesion is treated with pre-dilation using balloon angioplasty to create a larger lumen. Post-deployment angioplasty can be used to help the stent oppose the arterial wall (3).

Key Points

- Stenting is a technique that provides scaffolding for luminal expansion.
- Stenting is indicated for significant vessel stenosis or occlusion that cause various symptoms depending on the affected vasculature.
- Stents can be differentiated based on their composition material, design, deployment system, and drug elution properties.
- Complications of stenting include distal embolization, arterial trauma, and acute vessel occlusion.

References

1. Schillinger M, Sabeti S, Loewe C, et al. Balloon angioplasty versus implantation of nitinol stents in the superficial femoral artery.N Engl J Med. 2006;354(18):1879–1888.
2. Pearce B, Jordan WJ Jr. Nonaortic stents and stent-grafts. Cronenwett JL, Johnston KW, eds. Rutherford's Vascular Surgery. 8th ed. Philadelphia: Elsevier Saunders; 2014. Vol 2: 1443–1455.
3. Sullivan TM, Rizvi AZ. Technique: endovascular therapeutic. Cronenwett JL, Johnston KW, eds. Rutherford's Vascular Surgery. 8th ed. Philadelphia: Elsevier Saunders; 2014. Vol 2: 1322–1337.
4. Duerig, Tom. Metals as Implantable Materials. nitinol.com/wp-content/uploads/references/Metals-as-Implantable-Materials.pdf.
5. Chu TM, Chan YC, Cheng SW. Evidence for treating peripheral arterial diseases with biodegradable scaffolds. J Cardiovasc Surg (Torino). 2017;58(1):87–94.
6. Antoniou GA, Chalmers N, Kanesalingham K, Antoniou SA, Schiro A, Serracino-Inglott F, et al. Meta-analysis of outcomes of endovascular treatment of infrapopliteal occlusive disease with drug-eluting stents. J Endovasc Ther. 2013;20(2):131–144.

CHAPTER 11

STENT GRAFTS

Ryan Moore, Matthew Janko, Vikram S. Kashyap

KEYWORDS

aneurysm, dissection, stent graft, endograft, endoprosthesis, EVAR, TEVAR, endoleak

LEARNING OBJECTIVES

- To identify the advantages and risks of endovascular stent grafts and their indications for use
- To identify the different types of stent grafts available
- To describe the fundamental technical principles of EVAR and TEVAR

Endovascular stent grafts are fabric tubes incorporated together with metal stents that are delivered within the lumen of a blood vessel. Stent grafts are typically used for treatment of aortic aneurysms or dissections (Figures 11.1, 11.2, 11.3). Other general indications for the use of stent grafts can be found in Table 11.1. Stent grafts are frequently called "endografts" and in order to be effective the endograft must provide an adequate seal against the target vessel(s) at both proximal and distal areas of apposition, or "landing zones." The effectiveness and durability of the repair relies on the quality and quantity of apposition at these sites. As such, there are anatomic characteristics that make success more likely (1, 2).

Characteristics of Aortic Stent Grafts

Graft fabric materials are made of either polytetrafluoroethylene (PTFE) or woven polyester fabric (i.e., Dacron). The degree of structural support from the stent component varies across devices. The stent may be situated within the graft material (endoskeleton) or outside of the graft material (exoskeleton). Stents are usually made of nitinol, stainless steel, or cobalt-chromium alloy, with nitinol being the most widely used. Most endografts are magnetic resonance imaging (MRI) compatible, but individual safety and manufacturing information must be reviewed carefully prior to MRI or similar procedure.

Aortic endografts are typically deployed via the femoral arteries and are fixed proximally and distally to a non-aneurysmal aorta or iliac segments, excluding an aneurysm sac from the circulation. The endovascular abdominal aneurysm repair (EVAR) and thoracic stent graft (thoracic endovascular aortic repair [TEVAR]) techniques have been shown to be associated with decreased perioperative morbidity and mortality (1). Along with a minimally invasive approach, other advantages to the technique include shorter hospitalization often without the need for intensive care, decreased postoperative pain, and the ability to use regional or epidural anesthesia.

There are numerous endograft systems available in the United States, and new designs and delivery systems are constantly being tested. Despite their differences in design, three core design components are shared among endograft device systems:

1. **Delivery System:** Typically, the endograft is delivered via the femoral arteries either percutaneously or by direct surgical cutdown (3, 4). If femoral vessels are not suitable for use, an iliac exposure and conduit may be required (5).
2. **Main Body Device:** The largest portion of the endograft is deployed to a position that is usually below the renal arteries but occasionally above the renal arteries if a fenestrated or branched complex endograft is being used to maintain perfusion to the aortic branch arteries.
3. **Extensions:** One or more extension stent grafts that insert into the main body to complete the repair.

Endovascular Abdominal Aortic Repair

Anatomic eligibility for EVAR is mainly based on three areas:

1. **Infra-Renal Proximal Landing Zone ("Aortic Neck")**
   a. **Diameter:** The aortic diameter near the lowest renal artery.

b. **Length:** The distance from the lowest renal artery to the origin of the aneurysm.

c. **Angulation:** The angle formed between points connecting the proximal aorta, the middle of the aneurysm, and the aortic bifurcation.

2. **Distal Landing Zone:** The routine distal landing zones for stent graft extension modular components are the common iliac arteries. Occasionally the aneurysm may involve the common iliac and/or internal iliac arteries, and these may need to be excluded from the circulation. If this occurs, sacrifice of the ipsilateral internal artery or use of a specialized branched stent graft may be necessary in order to land in a non-aneurysmal artery segment.

3. **Access Arteries:** A minimal external iliac artery diameter of 7 mm is needed to allow safe passage of most delivery sheaths.

Some aneurysms are located very close to the renal arteries, providing insufficient space for an appropriate sealing zone at the proximal end of the graft without covering the renal arteries. This is called a **juxtarenal aortic aneurysm**. These aneurysms require a **fenestrated or branched graft** in which there are openings in the sides of the graft exactly where it should land over the renal and visceral arteries.

Procedure

The steps and materials required for EVAR placement using a standard modular device are as follows:

1. **Vessel access** is obtained by percutaneous (closure device) or open (surgical instruments) approach.

2. **Systemic anticoagulation** is initiated prior to device insertion, most often using intravenous heparin with a target activated clotting time (ACT) of 300 or twice the patient's baseline. After deployment, anticoagulation may or may not be reversed.

3. **Aortic angiography** is obtained by placing a pigtail catheter in the visceral aorta over a Glidewire. A power injector is required to opacify the aorta with contrast (Figure 11.4). Appropriate imaging angulation must be employed to correct for parallax. Preoperative cross-sectional imaging may be used at this step, if available.

4. **Main aortic endograft deployment** is accomplished over a heavy support wire. Any associated renal or visceral stents are also deployed at this time if appropriate.

5. The **contralateral iliac artery stent graft "gate" is cannulated** using a Glidewire. This step is confirmed by rotating a pigtail catheter into the main aortic endograft and rotating the catheter to ensure unencumbered free rotation, or by angiography.

6. **Length measurements** are obtained using marker catheters and angiography, and **extension stent grafts are deployed** using a heavy support wire. Again, correct angulation must be employed to ensure adequate visualization of the iliac artery bifurcation.

7. The **stent grafts are expanded** to their full diameter using a compliant balloon, followed by completion angiography (Figure 11.5) to assess for branch artery patency or complication (described later in the chapter). The **device sheaths are then removed** and the arteriotomies are closed either primarily or with percutaneous closure devices.

Thoracic Endovascular Aortic Repair

TEVAR is a minimally invasive procedure to repair the thoracic aorta. At present, endograft placement in the ascending aorta and aortic arch are not routinely performed. The anatomic factors that must be taken into account when considering TEVAR are similar to EVAR planning but include features unique to the thoracic aorta:

1. **Aortic arch and descending thoracic aorta:** Routine preoperative evaluation of the thoracic aorta with computed tomography angiography (CTA) or other modalities involves assessment of the following:
   a. Endoluminal diameter of the proximal and distal seal zones; a 2-cm proximal seal zone is required for currently available thoracic stent grafts.
   b. Length of aortic coverage required.
   c. Degree of angulation and tortuosity.
   d. Any intraluminal thrombus or calcification.

2. **Access arteries:** Similar to EVAR, femoral and iliac vessels that are not suitable for passage of an endograft may require direct retroperitoneal access, usage of an iliac conduit, or other special maneuvers.

3. **Neuroprotection:** Spinal cord ischemia is perhaps the most devastating complication of TEVAR, occurring in 0–13% of patients (11). Cerebrospinal fluid drainage using a lumbar spinal catheter ("lumbar drain") is often used to mitigate the risk of

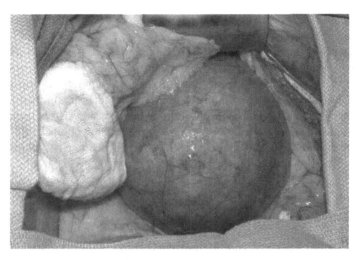

Figure 11.1 Abdominal aortic aneurysm.

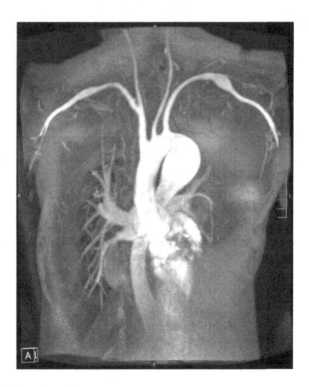

Figure 11.2 Thoracic aortic aneurysm.

neurological insult by decreasing pressure in the subarachnoid space and increasing perfusion.

4. **Debranching:** It is critical to note if the intended aortic stent graft coverage involves any of the aortic arch vessels or mesenteric vessels. If so, open debranching bypass may need to be considered prior to TEVAR. Open techniques such as ascending aorta-innominate, ascending aortic-left common carotid, and left carotid-subclavian bypasses are typical. Endovascular alternatives to debranching procedures include the use of "snorkeled" grafts as well as fenestrated grafts similar to those used in EVAR.

Postoperative Care and Surveillance

The majority of patients can be discharged home within the first 24 hours after EVAR. Peripheral pulses should be regularly assessed and compared with preoperative and immediate postoperative exams. Fluid resuscitation is key to avoid contrast nephropathy. Patients should resume their normal medications as appropriate. CTA is recommended at follow-up intervals (e.g., within 3–6 months postoperatively, followed by repeat CTA annually and/ or alternating with duplex ultrasonography) (7). Type I and III endoleaks after TEVAR require definitive management, while type II endoleaks require intervention if associated with aneurysm expansion.

Table 11.1 General Indications for Stent Graft Use

Indication	Example Target Vessel	Criteria
Aneurysm	Aorta	Diameter >5.5 cm; growth of 5 mm per 6 months or 10 mm per year
	Popliteal artery	Diameter >2 cm; association with thromboembolism
Dissection	Aorta	Malperfusion or other symptoms; aortic intramural hematoma (AIH) depth >14 mm; penetrating aortic ulcer (PAU) diameter or depth >2 cm
Blunt Injury	Aorta, often immediately distal to left subclavian artery after motor vehicle trauma	Grade III (pseudoaneurysm) or IV (transection) injury
Fistula	Aortoenteric, aortocaval, iliac artery to ureter	Typically performed to stabilize patients until definitive repair can be performed

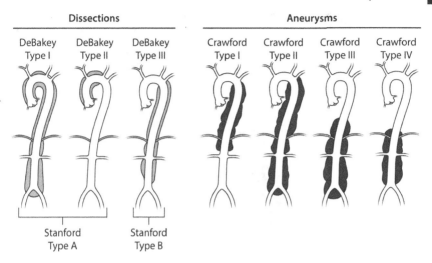

Dissections			Aneurysms			
DeBakey Type I	DeBakey Type II	DeBakey Type III	Crawford Type I	Crawford Type II	Crawford Type III	Crawford Type IV

Stanford Type A · Stanford Type B

Figure 11.3 DeBakey classification and Crawford classification for aortic dissections and aortic aneurysms.

Complications

The incidence of complications following EVAR is between 11% and 30% (6). The need for secondary intervention is common, carrying a yearly risk of approximately 10–15% (6).

1. **Access site complications** occur in 9% to 16% of patients (6) and include groin hematoma, acute arterial thrombosis, dissection, pseudoaneurysm, arteriovenous fistula, and distal embolization.
2. **Endoleak** is defined as a persistent flow of blood into the aneurysm sac after deployment of the graft, indicating a failure to completely exclude the aneurysm (8). Diagnosis is usually made using arteriography or ultrasound and is associated with a risk for aneurysm expansion and rupture. Endoleaks are classified as type I through IV based on the location of the leak (Figure 11.6).
3. **Device migration** is caused by proximal aortic neck dilation. If untreated this may lead to endoleak, aneurysm expansion, and rupture.
4. **Separation of components, limb kinking, and occlusion** are uncommon due to modular stent graft design (9). These

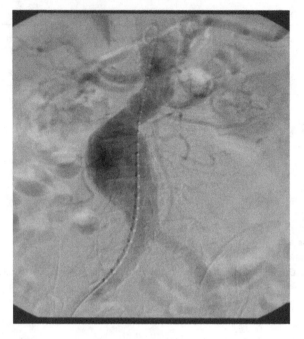

Figure 11.4 Aortogram before EVAR.

complications can be diagnosed by CTA or ultrasound and are
repaired by placing a bridging stent or converting to an aorto-uni-iliac
graft.

5. **Endograft infection** occurs in 0.4–3% of patients and is associated
   with a mortality rate between 25% and 50% (10). Conservative
   management is based on antibiotic therapy, while aggressive
   approaches favor surgical removal with immediate aortic
   reconstruction.
6. **Ischemia** may occur at the extremities, intestines, pelvis, kidney,
   and/or spine (11). These complications can be secondary to
   technical aspects of graft placement in relation to normal anatomic
   blood supply or from thromboembolic complications related to
   anticoagulation.
7. **Post-implantation syndrome** is defined as fever and leukocytosis
   associated with pleural effusion with an otherwise negative infectious
   workup. This is a benign phenomenon related to inflammation after
   graft placement and requires no intervention.

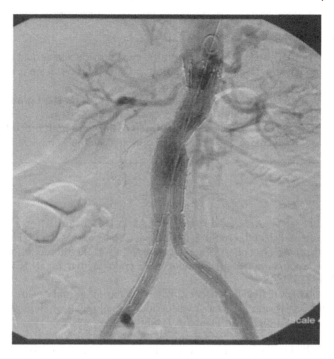

Figure 11.5 Aortogram after EVAR.

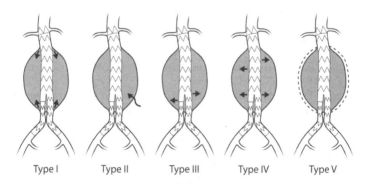

Type I   Type II   Type III   Type IV   Type V

Figure 11.6 Endoleaks.

Key Points

- Stent grafts, also known as endografts, must provide an adequate seal against the target vessel(s) at both proximal and distal areas of apposition, known as "landing zones."
- EVAR and TEVAR are two of the most common uses for stent grafts and may be utilized for aneurysmal or occlusive vascular disease.
- It is essential to be familiar with each step of the stent graft procedures in order to decrease the likelihood of potentially lethal complications.

References

1. Lin PH, et al. Arterial disease. In: Charles Brunicardi F, et al., editors. Schwartz's Principles of Surgery. 11th ed. New York: McGraw-Hill; 2019.
2. Schanzer A, Greenberg RK, Hevelone N, et al. Predictors of abdominal aortic aneurysm sac enlargement after endovascular repair. Circulation. 2011; 123:2848.
3. Howell M, Villareal R, Krajcer Z. Percutaneous access and closure of femoral artery access sites associated with endoluminal repair of abdominal aortic aneurysms. J Endovasc Ther. 2001; 8:68.
4. Nelson PR, Kracjer Z, Kansal N, et al. A multicenter, randomized, controlled trial of totally percutaneous access versus open femoral exposure for endovascular aortic aneurysm repair (the PEVAR trial). J Vasc Surg. 2014;59:1181.
5. Abu-Ghaida AM, Clair DG, Greenberg RK, et al. Broadening the applicability of endovascular aneurysm repair: the use of iliac conduits. J Vasc Surg. 2002;36:111.
6. Nordon IM, Karthikesalingam A, Hinchliffe RJ, et al. Secondary interventions following endovascular aneurysm repair (EVAR) and the enduring value of graft surveillance. Eur J Vasc Endovasc Surg. 2010;39:547.
7. Zaiem F, Almasri J, Tello M, Prokop LJ, Chaikof EL, Murad MH. A systematic review of surveillance after endovascular aortic repair. J Vasc Surg. 2018;67(1):320–331.
8. Gleason TG. Endoleaks after endovascular aortic stent-grafting: impact, diagnosis, and management. Semin Thorac Cardiovasc Surg. 2009;21:363.
9. England A, McWillians R. Migration and dislocation of aortic devices during follow-up. In: Branchereau A, Jacobs M, editors. Endovascular Aortic Repair: The State of the Art. Rome: Minerva Medica; 2008.
10. Smeds MR, Duncan AA, Harlander-Locke MP, et al. Treatment and outcomes of aortic endograft infection. J Vasc Surg. 2016;63:332.
11. Ullery BW, Cheung AT, Fairman RM, et al. Risk factors, outcomes, and clinical manifestations of spinal cord ischemia following thoracic endovascular aortic repair. J Vasc Surg. 2011;54:677–684.

CHAPTER 12

ATHERECTOMY DEVICES

Saideep Bose, Mehdi Shishehbor

KEYWORDS

atherectomy, debulking, laser, orbital, directional, excisional, rotational, aspirational, vessel preparation

LEARNING OBJECTIVES

- When is atherectomy a useful adjunct to traditional angioplasty/stenting?
- Which atherectomy devices are best suited for a particular lesion?

The main concept behind atherectomy is modifying and debulking atherosclerotic lesions. This is in contrast to angioplasty and stenting, which generally leave the existing disease in place and focus on improving luminal gain.

One of the problems with balloon angioplasty, especially in heavily calcified lesions, is that there is significant recoil associated with the underlying bulky plaque. Although there may be significant luminal gain on an angiogram after initial balloon dilation, the vessel may recoil to its initial diameter or smaller soon thereafter, especially if there is significant damage to the vessel associated with aggressive dilation. This recoil can partially be addressed with stents, which help to maintain luminal gain. However, stents have their share of downsides: they are more prone to fracture/kinking at sites of high mechanical stress (common in a flexible, dynamic vessel such as the superficial femoral artery), and they cannot be used in junctional areas where there is a bifurcation or a trifurcation without potentially "jailing" an important vessel. Furthermore, in some cases, complete thrombosis of the stent and the underlying vessel can lead to more severe ischemia than the initial presentation. In addition, overaggressive stenting may compromise future surgical bypass targets in a patient.

With all this being said, atherectomy is rarely used alone and instead is used as adjunctive therapy with angioplasty and stenting. The rationale is that atherectomy can straighten eccentric lesions and debulk heavily calcified ones so that the native lumen is widened and overstretching with balloon angioplasty can be avoided. Stenting is then used selectively when there is a significant residual stenosis or a hemodynamically significant dissection.

Types of Devices

Currently approved atherectomy devices can be grouped into their mechanisms of action: rotational, orbital, directional, and photo-ablative (Table 12.1). There are generally multiple different vendors of each type of device, but the principles behind each category are the same (Figure 12.1). Each device has studies demonstrating safety of use and clinical effectiveness. However, there are no large-scale studies that have compared the devices head to head in the peripheral vasculature to objectively determine which atherectomy method may be better for a given location and type of lesion.

Rotational

Jetstream (Boston Scientific). Rotational devices such as this one have rotating cutting blades near the tip of the catheter that act like a drill through lesions. This specific device has an aspiration system built in proximal to the tip that allows it to continually evacuate the debunked debris. The system works through a 7Fr sheath and over a 0.014″ wire.

Orbital

Diamondback 360 (CSI). The mechanism behind this device is using a diamond-coated sander that is eccentrically mounted on a wire so when the wire rotates, the sander "shaves" off calcium and plaque from the surrounding walls. The size of the luminal gain can be adjusted by increasing the speed of device. The system works through a 5 to 6Fr sheath over a 0.014″ wire.

Directional

HawkOne (Medtronic). This device has a slight bend at the distal end of the catheter, which opposes the cutting mechanism to one of the four quadrants

Table 12.1 Examples of Commercially Available Atherectomy Devices in Each Mechanistic Category (1)

Device Name	Mechanism of Action	Features	Working Length (cm)	Sheath Compatibility (Fr)
Jetstream	Rotational/ aspirational	Can be used for atherectomy and thrombectomy; front and differential cutting	120, 135, 145	7, 8
Diamondback 360	Orbital	Bidirectional eccentric crown designed to create concentric lumen. Plaque modification. Front cutting. Available in 145- and 60-cm shafts	160	4
SilverHawk/ TurboHawk	Directional/ excisional	Treat eccentric disease to maximize lumen gain	110, 113, 133, 135, 149	6-8
Excimer laser	Photo- ablative	May be used for total occlusion, in-stent restenosis, thrombus- containing lesions, soft plaques, and fibrous caps. Three different mechanisms of reducing plaque: chemical, thermal, and mechanical	110, 120, 130, 150	4-8

of the vessel. The rotating blade then shaves the plaque and packs it into the nose cone of the catheter, which must be periodically emptied throughout the procedure. The tip of the catheter may be rotated as necessary in multiple passes to cover all quadrants of the lumen. The system works over through a 6Fr or 7Fr sheath and over a 0.014″ wire. One benefit of this system is that it is self-contained and does not require any fixed capitol to operate. However, it is recommended that the system be used with a distal embolic protection device such as the SpiderFX.

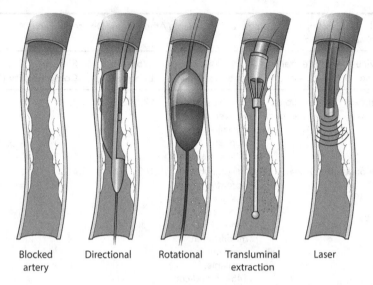

Figure 12.1 Side-by-side comparison of different atherectomy devices in plaque removal.

Photo-Ablative

Turbo-Elite (Spectranetics). The principal of the photo-ablative systems is to use light to vaporize tissue. By using short pulses, the energy is focused only on tissues that are within 50 μm of the tip, limiting damage to the native artery. The system works through a 4F to an 8F sheath over a 0.014–0.018″ wire.

When to Use Which Device

Oftentimes the choice of which atherectomy device to use is dictated by institutional availability and local practice, especially since many devices require up-front capital expenditure for generators or other reusable components. However, the general principle is that rotational devices may be better suited toward highly calcific lesions or chronic total occlusions, directional devices for eccentric lesions or soft plaque, and photo-ablative devices for in-stent restenosis and thrombus (Table 12.2).

Depending on the lesion that is treated, many centers now combine the use of atherectomy with drug-coated angioplasty or stenting to maximize patency. Furthermore, recent atherectomy devices such as the Pantheris (Avinger) combine an existing technology, in this case directional atherectomy, with built-in image guidance. It is yet to be seen whether this will lead to better outcomes in comparison with the existing atherectomy devices.

Table 12.2 Comparison of Scenarios Using Different Atherectomy Devices (2)

Atherectomy Type	Rotational	Directional	Photo-ablative
Eccentric lesion	+	++	
Soft/fibrotic plaque	++	++	++
Thrombotic lesion	+		+
Highly calcific lesion	++	+	+
Chronic total occlusion (CTO)	++	++	++
In-stent restenosis	+		++
In-stent occlusion with thrombosis	+		++

+ Effective
++ Highly effective

Summary

There is limited level 1 data on the efficacy of atherectomy devices for lower extremity intervention. Given the cost and lack of randomized data, these devices should be used judiciously. The use of embolic protection devices is likely necessary for most atherectomy cases. Furthermore, technical knowledge is critical in performing appropriate cases and atherectomy devices.

Key Points

- Atherectomy devices are a useful adjunct to modify lesions to minimize the need for bailout stenting.
- No randomized data exist to suggest which atherectomy devices are better in a given clinical context. The use of atherectomy devices is currently more driven by institutional availability and operator preference.

References

1. Shishehbor MH, Jaff MR. Percutaneous therapies for peripheral artery disease. Circulation. 2016;134(24):2008–2027.
2. Sunderdiek U. Experience with atherectomy and DCBs: the merits of a two-part approach in the SA and popliteal artery. In: Endovascular Today [Internet]. 2017. Available from: https://evtoday.com/articles/2017-sept-supplement2/experience-with-atherectomy-and-dcbs

CHAPTER 13

INTRAVASCULAR IMAGING MODALITIES (OCT AND IVUS)

Elder Iarossi Zago, Gabriel Tensol Rodriguez Pereira, Hiram Bezerra

KEYWORDS

OCT, IVUS, intravascular imaging, axial imaging

LEARNING OBJECTIVES

- Understand the basics of intravascular imaging devices and acquisition
- Understand the different capabilities and applications of intravascular imaging modalities
- Assess basic composition and morphology of different vascular lesions under IVUS and OCT

Although catheter-based angiography is the method used by most endovascular interventionalists to assess the severity and morphology of vascular lesions and guide treatment, it has many known limitations. Primarily, these images are lumenograms, depicting a two-dimensional projection of a contrast-filled lumen, with little information about the vessel wall and the vessel's inherent three-dimensional characteristics. Intravascular imaging—intravascular ultrasound (IVUS) and optical coherence tomography (OCT)—includes imaging modalities that utilize catheter-mounted probes to provide an axial cross-sectional image of a vessel to address the limitations of conventional angiography in imaging and interventions (1–4).

Clinical Applications

It is important to note that OCT and IVUS are often not interchangeable, nor are they routinely used to image the same vasculature. The different uses for these imaging catheters are largely a product of the capabilities and limitations provided to them by physics. These devices acquire images of a vessel in two very different manners: OCT with near-infrared light (900–1300 nm wavelength) and IVUS with ultrasonic frequency (10–40 MHz) sound waves. Both modalities are useful in morphologic assessment of vascular lesions, intervention guidance (lesion preparation, measurement of vessel dimensions and device selection, stent optimization), and assessment of culprit lesions (5–7).

The scenarios in which OCT are valuable are those in which the interventionalist is evaluating and treating complex intimal lesions in small vessels (2–5 mm) and where a high degree of accuracy is desired (e.g., coronary vasculature). This is because of the use of near-infrared light in OCT imaging, which conveys superior tissue resolution over IVUS (10 vs. 100 μm), but at the cost of reduced penetration into vessel walls (2 mm) (8, 9) (Table13.1). Therefore, OCT cannot be used to image larger vessels (e.g., aorta or vena cava) or accurately illuminate lesions involving deeper layers of a vessel. In addition, OCT requires the blood in the vessel to be displaced for imaging. This is usually done with contrast, which limits the size and number of

Table 13.1 Comparison of OCT and IVUS

	OCT	IVUS
Source of image	Near-infrared light	Ultrasound (10–40 MHz)
Blood clearance	Contrast 10–15 mL	Not required
Acquisition speedy	25 mm/s	0.5 mm/s
Pullback length	54–75 mm	Unlimited
Vessel size	2–5 mm	Up to 20 mm
Penetration depth	2 mm	4–8 mm
Axial resolution	10–20 μm	100–150 μm
Lateral resolution	20 μm	200 μm
Minimal guide catheter size	5Fr (although 6Fr preferable)	5Fr
Severity of calcium	Very good	Good
Lipid	Good detection, poor penetration	Good penetration, poor detection
Stent length	Very good	Very good
Stent sizing by vessel wall	Good	Very good
Stent malapposition	Very good	Good
Stent edge dissection	Very good	Good
Neoatherosclerosis	Very good	Good

vessels that can be imaged. The superior tissue resolution for which OCT is lauded allows it to reliably assess and quantify atherosclerotic plaque characteristics (thin fibrous cap, thrombus, neovessels, lipid pool, foamy macrophages) and differentiate early from advanced lesions, with close correlation with pathology. For this reason, OCT is primarily utilized in percutaneous coronary interventions (PCIs), but has some adoption among interventionalists across fields in evaluating and treating other small-vessel pathologies (e.g., atherosclerotic tibial disease).

IVUS enjoys use across interventional disciplines and in treating a wide range of pathologies. First pioneered in coronary interventions, IVUS use has expanded outward to be used extensively in aortic and large venous interventions (e.g., vena cava and iliac). The primary advantage of IVUS is its superior tissue penetration abilities (4–8 mm) and ability to image larger and longer vessels such as the aorta and vena cava. Despite this, its tissue resolution pales in comparison with OCT, making the workflow different between them: the blood displacement paired with OCT high resolution allows automatic vessel segmentation, whereas IVUS cross-sectional area should be traced manually (10–12).

Image Acquisition

IVUS

In general, IVUS catheters can be utilized in a live-imaging fashion or in a formal, pullback image acquisition approach. In the live-imaging fashion, the catheter is activated and advanced or withdrawn by the operator to view a live feed of vessel images. Pullback image acquisition functions to allow the device to capture and save a series of images either to be viewed in playback later, or to build a tomographic projection of a lesion or vessel; it can be performed manually or via automated, motorized functions where the device is withdrawn by an apparatus at a set speed. Manual transducer pullback should be performed slowly, at a rate similar to motorized pullback (speed of 0.5 mm/s). Advantages are the ability to concentrate on specific regions of interest by pausing the transducer motion at a specific location in the vessel. Disadvantages include the possibility of skipping over significant pathology by pulling the transducer too quickly or unevenly and the inability to perform precise length and volumetric measurements (12, 13). Philips and Boston Scientific are the key players in this market (Figure 13.1).

OCT

The OCT catheter is first advanced over a regular guidewire, distally to the region of interest. The second radiopaque marker, located right proximally to the OCT lens, can be used as a reference to place the catheter. Image acquisition is performed via an automated pullback method (similar to that of IVUS), and it requires a bolus of contrast material to be injected through the catheter to

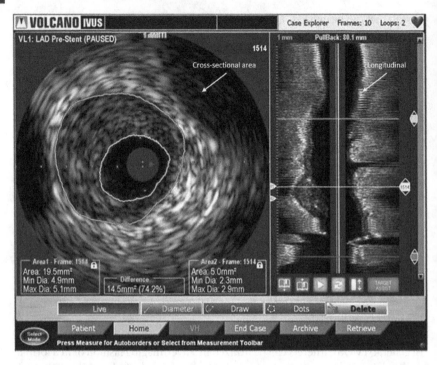

Figure 13.1 IVUS interface.

displace blood within the vessel and away from the view of the imaging probe. Because the wavelength of light utilized (900–1300 nm) is much smaller than the size of a red blood cell (6–8 μm), the presence of blood results in significant scattering of light; therefore, little returns back to the probe for image formation. The acquisition speed can range between 5 and 40 mm/s, based on the OCT system used and the pullback mode. Most expert users advocate the use of automated contrast injection to optimize the image quality (9). Current practice requires that the patients are anticoagulated, typically with heparin, before inserting the guidewire into the vessel. If it is not contraindicated, image acquisition should be conducted after the administration of intra-arterial nitroglycerin to minimize the potential for catheter-induced vasospasm (8, 14–16).

The main OCT manufacturers are Abbott and Terumo (not U.S. Food and Drug Administration approved) (Figure 13.2). Dragonfly™ OPTIS™ catheter (Abbott, see below) has three radiopaque markers. The first one is located distally (4 mm from the catheter tip), and the second marker is 23 mm from the first. This is important because this is where the OCT lens is. From that point proximally is the region that is going to be imaged. The third marker is 50 mm from the second marker.

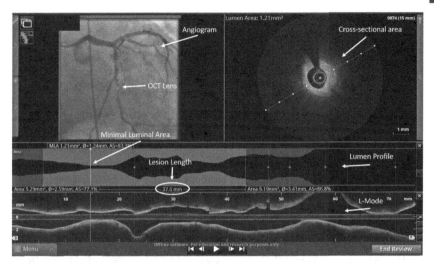

Figure 13.2 OCT interface: pre-PCI pullback.

OCT Acquisition Mnemonic: "4 Ps":

- Position – Ensure your target segment is between the lens and proximal markers.
- Purge – Clear the blood from the catheter lumen, if present.
- Puff – Inject a small amount of flush media through the guide catheter, during live view, to ensure you are obtaining adequate clearance.
- Pullback – Enable the beginning of the imaging process.

Fundamental OCT Language:

- **Backscatter**
  The reflection of the light waves off the tissue back to the lens.
  High backscatter means a brighter pixel; described as a "signal-rich" region.
  Low backscatter means a darker pixel; described as a "signal-poor" region.
- **Attenuation**
  The reduction in intensity of the light waves as they pass through tissue.
  High attenuation means the light cannot penetrate very deep.
  Low attenuation means the light can pass through to allow visualization of deeper tissue.

Fundamental IVUS Language:

- **Echogenic**
  The return echoes making it visible on the monitor.
- **Echolucent**
  Absence of echoes return, corresponding to black spaces on the monitor.

113

Image Interpretation

- **Normal or Non-Disease Vessel Anatomy** (Figure 13.3):
  a. **OCT:** The three layers (adventitia, media, and intima) of the artery are mostly visible. The media appears as a slightly darker band than the others two layers.
  b. **IVUS:** In the normal artery, two such interfaces are usually observed, one at the border between blood and the leading edge of the intima and a second at the external elastic membrane (EEM), which is located at the media-adventitia border. The intima is thin, consisting mostly of endothelial cells and connective tissue, with a relatively small difference in impedance from blood.
- **Abnormal** (Figure 13.4): A and A' represent fibrous plaque on OCT and IVUS, respectively. B and B' represent calcium. C and C' are lipid plaque, and D and D' show a dissection.
- **IVUS for Large-Vessel Pathology** (Figure 13.5): Example of the unique role IVUS plays in imaging large-vessel pathologies, such as those of the aorta and iliac veins. A and A' demonstrate a type B aortic dissection before and after thoracic endovascular aortic repair (TEVAR) placement (IVUS catheter probe located within the true lumen).
- **Malapposition** (Figure 13.6): For OCT and IVUS there is a lack of contact between stent struts and vessel wall. It is important to consider the stent thickness when making this assessment because the back edges of the struts are not visible on both methods.

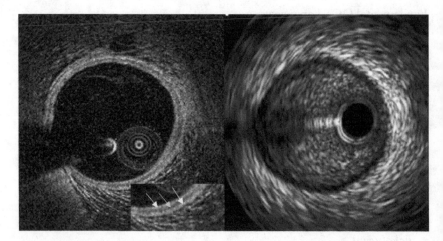

Figure 13.3 Outlay of normal vessel anatomy under OCT versus IVUS.

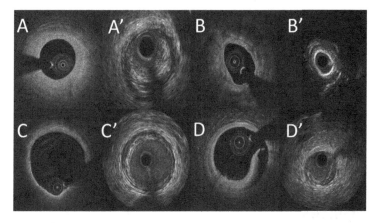

Figure 13.4 Comparison of various arterial pathologies under OCT versus IVUS.

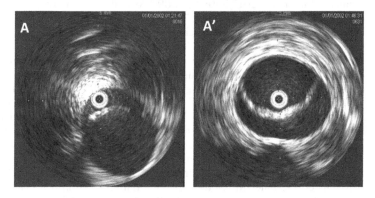

Figure 13.5 Aortic dissection pre- and post-TEVAR deployment.

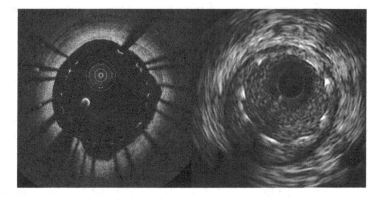

Figure 13.6 Stent malapposition as visualized under OCT versus IVUS.

Key Points

- Intravascular imaging provides detailed and accurate measurements of vessel lumen morphology, vessel size, extension of diseased artery segments, and vessel size and plaque characteristics.
- OCT conveys superior tissue resolution over IVUS but at the cost of reduced penetration into vessel walls, the need to displace blood for imaging, and inability to image large vessels.
- The principal clinical applications for IVUS/OCT are guiding interventions and clarifying ambiguous or indeterminate radiograph angiography.

References

1. Mintz GS, Guagliumi G. Intravascular imaging in coronary artery disease. Lancet. [Internet]. 2017;390:793–809. Available from: http://dx.doi.org/10.1016/S0140-6736(17)31957-8

2. Huang D, Swanson EA, Lin CP, Schuman JS, Stinson WG, Chang W, et al. Optical coherence tomography. Science. 1991;254(5035):1178–1181.

3. Brezinski ME, Tearney GJ, Bouma BE, Izatt JA, Hee MR, Swanson EA, et al. Optical coherence tomography for optical biopsy: properties and demonstration of vascular pathology. Circulation. 1996;93(6):1206–1213.

4. Levine GN, Bates ER, Blankenship JC, Bailey SR, Bittl JA, Cercek B, et al. ACCF/AHA/SCAI Practice Guideline 2011 ACCF/AHA/SCAI Guideline for Percutaneous Coronary Intervention: Executive summary a report of the American College of Cardiology Foundation/American Heart Association Task Force on Practice Guidelines and the Society for Cardiovascular Angiography and Interventions. Circulation. 2011;124(23):2574–2609.

5. Adriaenssens T, Joner M, Godschalk TC, Malik N, Alfonso F, Xhepa E, et al. Optical coherence tomography findings in patients with coronary stent thrombosis. Circulation. 2017;136(11):1007–1021.

6. Mintz GS. Clinical utility of intravascular imaging and physiology in coronary artery disease. J Am Coll Cardiol. 2014;64(2):207–222.

7. Raber L, Brugaletta S, Yamaji K, O'Sullivan CJ, Otsuki S, Koppara T, et al. Very late scaffold thrombosis: intracoronary imaging and histopathological and spectroscopic findings. J Am Coll Cardiol. 2015;66(17):1901–1914.

8. Regar E, Akasaka T, Adriaenssens T, Barlis P, Bezerra HG, Bouma B, et al. Consensus Standards for Acquisition, Measurement, and Reporting of Intravascular Optical Coherence Tomography Studies: a report from the International Working Group for Intravascular Optical Coherence Tomography Standardization and Validation. J Am Coll Cardiol. 2012;59(12):1058–1072.

9. Prati F, Guagliumi G, Mintz GS, Costa M, Regar E, Akasaka T, et al. Expert Review Document Part 2 : Methodology, Terminology and Clinical Applications of Optical Coherence Tomography for the Assessment of Interventional Procedures. Eur Heart J. 2012;33(20):2513–2522.

10. McDaniel MC, Eshtehardi P, Sawaya FJ, Douglas Jr JS, Samady H. Contemporary clinical applications of coronary intravascular ultrasound. JACC Cardiovasc Interv. 2011;4(11):1155–1167.
11. Doyley M, Mastik F, Carlier S, Serruys PW. Advancing intravascular ultrasonic palpation toward clinical applications. Ultrasound Med Biol. 2001;27(11):1471–1480.
12. Nissen SE, Yock P. Intravascular ultrasound: novel pathophysiological insights and current clinical applications. Circulation. 2001;103(4):604–616.
13. Mintz GS, Nissen SE, Anderson W, Bailey SR, Erbel R, Fitzgerald PJ, et al. American College of Cardiology Clinical Expert Consensus Document on Standards for Acquisition, Measurement and Reporting of Intravascular Ultrasound Studies (IVUS). J Am Coll Cardiol. 2001;37(5):1478–1492.
14. Bezerra HG, Costa MA, Guagliumi G, Rollins A, Simon DI. Intracoronary optical coherence tomography: a comprehensive review of clinical research applications. JACC Cardiovasc Interv. 2009;2(11):1035–1046.
15. Barlis P, Schmitt J. Current and future developments in intracoronary optical coherence tomography imaging. EuroIntervention. 2009;4(4):529–533.
16. Katwal AB, Lopez JJ. Technical considerations and practical guidance for intracoronary optical coherence tomography. Interv Cardiol Clin. 2015;4(3):239–249.

CHAPTER 14

POST-PROCEDURAL HEMOSTASIS AND CLOSURE DEVICES

Cassandra Beck, Christopher Smolock

LEARNING OBJECTIVES

- Understand the methods of obtaining access site hemostasis
- Recognize factors to consider before pulling a sheath
- Know the technique of holding manual compression
- Become familiar with common vascular closure devices
- Appreciate advantages and limitations of each method of vascular closure

Access Site Management

Access-related complications are the most common complication of endovascular procedures (1). Obtaining hemostasis is best achieved when the access site is selected well and the puncture site is managed properly during and after the procedure (2). The common femoral artery is the most common vessel used to gain arterial access (3). Local vascular complications resulting from percutaneous access or closure may result in hematoma, pseudoaneurysm, dissection, or thrombosis (4).

The traditional method of closure is manual compression. This is performed with sustained pressure over the puncture site until hemostasis is achieved, followed by bed rest for 6 hours. Additional methods using vascular closure devices (VCDs) have been developed with the intent to minimize manual compression time and allow earlier return to ambulation. Deciding which method to use is patient and vessel specific and depends on caliber of the vessel, local vascular disease, size of arteriotomy, body habitus, scarring

Table 14.1 Comparison of Manual Compression and Vascular Closure Devices

Method	Benefit	Limitation
Manual compression	• Not limited to CFA access • No device cost • Heavily calcified vessel • Scarred groins • Prosthetic graft access	• Delayed ambulation • Patient discomfort • Time intensive • Not ideal for large sheaths > 7Fr • Difficult in obese groins • Requires anticoagulant reversal
Vascular closure devices	• Shortened hemostasis • Decreased time to ambulation • Less time intensive • Larger sheaths > 7Fr • Can be used with therapeutic anticoagulation or DAPT	• Requires technical expertise • Deployment or device failures • Limited to CFA access • Device cost • Increased risk of infection • Increased risk of limb ischemia

Abbreviations: CFA, Common femoral artery; DAPT, dual antiplatelet therapy.

around access site, and need for anticoagulation post-procedure. The benefits and limitations of each method of closure are listed in Table 14.1.

Successfully obtaining access site hemostasis at the completion of any procedure requires adequate preparation and technique (4). Factors to consider prior to sheath removal and vessel closure are patient comfort and ability to lay supine for a prolonged period of time, degree of anticoagulation, and blood pressure. Methods to address the above factors include administering additional local anesthetic or sedation, measuring the activated clotting time (ACT), giving protamine to reverse heparin, or administering antihypertensive medication.

Manual Compression

When manual pressure is chosen as the method of vascular closure, digital pressure is held until hemostasis is achieved. A general rule of thumb is to hold pressure for approximately 3 minutes per French size, for example, 18 minutes for a 6Fr sheath.

Prior to removing the sheath, assess the peripheral pulses and examine the access site for hematoma. Set the bed at an appropriate height to allow full arm extension and apply upper body weight if needed to hold firm pressure.

Remember that the arteriotomy will be 2–3 cm proximal to the skin entry site in most cases. Place the middle three fingers of the hand proximal to the sheath site. Remove the sheath slowly at the same angle at which it was inserted. Apply firm pressure over the arteriotomy site once the sheath has been removed. Care must be taken so that digital pressure does not occlude vessel flow but is firm enough to prevent bleeding from the arteriotomy. The pulse should be readily palpable while maintaining pressure until hemostasis is achieved. Bed rest is recommended for 6 hours with patient flat for the first hour then with head of the bed raised to 30 degrees for the remainder of bed rest.

Arterial Closure Devices

Alternative modes of obtaining hemostasis after percutaneous endovascular procedures are with VCDs. These devices have been shown to reduce time to hemostasis, facilitate earlier patient mobilization, and improve patient comfort (5–8). They have not been shown to decrease access site complications when compared with manual compression (5–8). Although rare, VCDs have been shown to increase the risk of leg ischemia, groin infection, and complications requiring surgical repair compared with manual compression (8).

VCDs use active or passive approximation for access site closure. Active devices physically close the arteriotomy with the use of a suture, nitinol clip, or collagen plug. Passive devices deploy an extraluminal sealant at the arteriotomy site without actively closing the arteriotomy. Ideally, a closure device should be simple to use, safe, reliable, and inexpensive. Currently available devices demonstrate strengths and weaknesses in each of these areas.

VCDs are indicated for both interventional and diagnostic procedures. VCDs may be especially desirable in situations where early ambulation is desired, in patients who require post-procedural anticoagulation, after thrombolytic therapy, in obese patients, or in procedures requiring large sheaths. Requirements for use of a VCD include common femoral access, minimal lumen diameter 4–6 mm (device specific), and absence of severe disease. If a VCD fails, manual compression can be used to achieve hemostasis. Open repair may be required for large arteriotomies or when vessel damage occurs.

Commonly selected devices are described and listed in Table 14.2. A more detailed description of individual devices and deployment methods can be found on each of the manufacturer's websites.

Perclose ProGlide (Abbott Vascular) actively approximates by deploying an arterial suture that exits percutaneously with a pre-tied knot on each side of

Table 14.2 Common Vascular Closure Device Specifications

Device	Manufacturer	Closure Method	Sheath Size (Fr)	Wire (inches)	Comments
Perclose ProGlide	Abbott Vascular	Active, suture	5–21	0.038	• >8Fr requires two devices and pre-close technique • Monofilament polypropylene suture with automatic knot formation • Maintains wire access
Prostar XL	Abbott Vascular	Active, suture	8.5–10	0.038	• Procedures requiring large sheaths • Two braided polyester sutures • Maintains wire access
StarClose	Abbott Vascular	Active Nitinol clip	5 6	0.038	• Extravascular permanent nitinol clip
AngioSeal	St. Jude Medical	Active Collagen plug	6 8	0.035 0.038	• Intravascular anchor secured to extravascular collagen plug with a suture • Bioabsorbable
Mynx	Cardinal Health/Cordis	Passive PEG sealant	5 6/7	0.038	• Polyethylene glycol extravascular sealant • Bioabsorbable • 5 min manual compression
Vascade	Cardiva Medical	Passive Collagen patch	5 6/7	0.038	• Extravascular thrombogenic collagen patch • Bioabsorbable • 5 min manual compression

the arteriotomy site (Figure 14.1). The arteriotomy is closed by tightening the suture loop. For sheaths >8Fr, two devices and a "pre-close" technique are required. The device can be used to "pre-close" large arteriotomies up to 21Fr before endovascular aneurysm repair (9). No additional manual compression required unless bleeding persists. Bed rest is recommended for 0–2 hours.

StarClose (Abbott Vascular) actively approximates by deploying a 4-mm extravascular nitinol clip over the arteriotomy site (Figure 14.2). The clip grasps the tissue on top of the artery around the access site in a purse-string

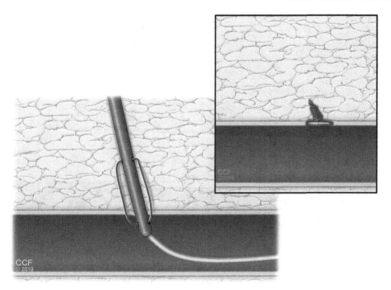

Figure 14.1 Perclose ProGlide, active closure device. A suture loop is formed and tightened to close the arteriotomy.

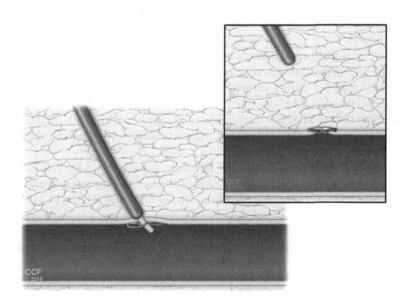

Figure 14.2 StarClose, active closure device. A 4-mm nitinol clip is deployed over the arteriotomy to close the media and adventitia.

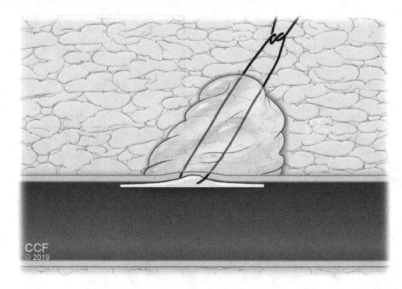

Figure 14.3 AngioSeal, active closure device. Absorbable intravascular anchor tethered to an extravascular collagen plug closes arteriotomy.

fashion designed to close the adventitia and media (9). No additional manual compression is required unless bleeding persists. Bed rest is recommended for 0–2 hours.

AngioSeal (St. Jude Medical) actively approximates the arteriotomy site by the use of an intravascular anchor and an extravascular collagen plug tethered together with a suture (Figure 14.3). The collagen plug facilitates coagulation, speeding up the process of hemostasis. All components, including the intravascular anchor, are fully resorbed within 60–90 days (9). No additional manual compression is required unless bleeding persists. Bed rest is recommended for 0–2 hours.

Mynx (Cardinal Health/Cordis) passively approximates by delivering a polyethylene glycol sealant to the extravascular space over the arteriotomy while a balloon occludes the arteriotomy from within the vessel (Figure 14.4). After deployment, the balloon is deflated and removed leaving only the expanded sealant, which securely adheres to the arteriotomy and dissolves within 30 days. Additional manual compression is required for up to 5 minutes or until hemostasis is achieved. Bed rest is recommended for 2–4 hours.

Vascade (Cardiva Medical) passively approximates by delivering an extravascular collagen patch over the arteriotomy while a conformable disc occludes the arteriotomy from within the vessel (Figure 14.5). After deployment, the disc is collapsed and the device is removed. The collagen patch

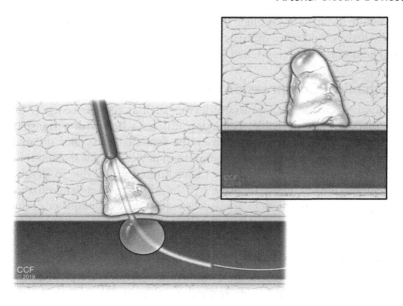

Figure 14.4 Mynx, passive closure device. Absorbable extravascular PEG sealant adheres to an arteriotomy.

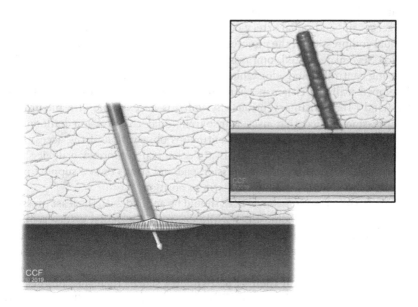

Figure 14.5 Vascade, passive closure device. Absorbable extravascular collagen patch expands to tamponade arteriotomy and promote hemostasis.

expands to mechanically occlude the tract and aid in hemostasis. It fully resorbs in 60–90 days. Additional manual compression is required for up to 5 minutes or until hemostasis is achieved. Bed rest is recommended for 2–4 hours.

Mechanical Compression Devices

External mechanical compression devices such as the FemoStop (Abbott Vascular) are also available. FemoStop utilizes a belt with a transparent pneumatic dome that is placed over the femoral artery and inflated to achieve hemostasis. Mechanical compression devices do not shorten time to hemostasis or ambulation and often have limited utility due to significant patient discomfort when in place (5). In addition, close surveillance is necessary to ensure the device has not inadvertently dislodged or occluded the femoral artery.

Radial Access Closure

Transradial access for diagnostic or interventional coronary procedures has now been adopted as the preferred access site approach as well as a viable alternative to femoral access for some peripheral vascular procedures. The superficial position of the radial artery and ease of compression reduce the risk of access site complications compared with femoral artery access (10, 11). The primary objectives of radial artery hemostasis are to prevent bleeding from the access site and radial artery occlusion. This can be achieved by applying manual compression at the puncture site or by using a mechanical hemostasis device. Several dedicated compression devices, most in the form of wristbands exerting controlled and adjustable pressure over the radial artery, have been developed utilizing either mechanical or pneumatic compression (12). The TR Band (Terumo Interventional Systems) is an example of a pneumatic compression device that uses transparent dual compression balloons to provide precise compression and continuous observation of the access site. The RadiStop (Abbott Vascular) is a mechanical compression device that incorporates a transparent compression pad and straps onto a support plate that holds the hand, wrist, and forearm in position.

Radial artery compression devices should be applied with the least pressure necessary to achieve hemostasis while ensuring the radial artery remains patent. This can be tested by applying a pulse oximetry probe to the index finger of the involved hand and occluding the ipsilateral ulnar artery manually. If the oximetry signal remains present, then patent hemostasis has been achieved successfully. If there is no oximetry signal, then the compression device can be gradually loosened until the signal returns. The device is removed, on average, after 2–3 hours. Close surveillance is required while the device is in place.

Key Points

- Access site hemostasis can be achieved by manual compression or with the use of a VSD.
- Patient comfort, degree of anticoagulation, and blood pressure are factors to consider prior to pulling a sheath.
- Manual compression is performed by applying digital pressure with the middle three fingers proximal to skin entry site with enough force to prevent bleeding without occluding vessel flow.
- Active VCDs physically close the arteriotomy with use of a suture (Perclose ProGlide), nitinol clip (StarClose), or collagen plug (AngioSeal). Passive VCDs deploy a PEG sealant (Mynx) or collagen patch (Vascade) to extravascular space without physically closing the arteriotomy.
- Manual compression may be preferred for diagnostic procedures, small sheath sizes, heavily calcified access vessels, scarred groins, or when prosthetic graft is accessed. VCDs may be preferred when instant hemostasis and early ambulation is desired, for large arteriotomies, when post-procedure anticoagulation or dual antiplatelet therapy (DAPT) is required, or for obese groins where manual compression may be difficult.

References

1. Siracuse JJ, Menard MT, Eslami MH, Kalish JA, Robinson WP, Eberhardt RT, et al. Comparison of open and endovascular treatment of patients with critical limb ischemia in the Vascular Quality Initiative. J. Vasc. Surg. 2016;63(4):958–965.
2. Lo RC, Fokkema MTM, Curran T, Darling J, Hamdan AD, Wyers M, et al. Routine use of ultrasound-guided access reduces access site-related complications after lower extremity percutaneous revascularization. J Vasc Surg. 2015;61(2):405–412.
3. DeRubertis BG, Faries PL, McKinsey JF, Chaer RA, Pierce M, Karwowski J, et al. Shifting paradigms in the treatment of lower extremity vascular disease: a report of 1000 percutaneous interventions. Ann Surg. 2007; 246(3):415–422.
4. Hackl G, Gary T, Belaj K, Hafner F, Eller P, Brodmann M. Risk factors for puncture site complications after endovascular procedures in patients with peripheral arterial disease. Vasc Endovascular Surg. 2015;49(7):160–165.
5. Robertson L, Andras A, Colgan F, Jackson R. Vascular closure devices for femoral arterial puncture site haemostasis. Cochrane Database of Systematic Reviews. 2016;3:CD009541.
6. Vaitkus PT. A meta-analysis of percutaneous vascular closure devices after diagnostic catheterization and percutaneous coronary intervention. J Invasive Cardiol. 2004;16(5):243–246.

7. Nikolsky E, Mehran R, Halkin A, Aymong ED, Mintz GS, Lasic Z, et al. Vascular complications associated with arteriotomy closure devices in patients undergoing percutaneous coronary procedures: a meta-analysis. J Am Coll Cardiol. 2004;44(6):1200–1209.

8. Biancari F, D'Andrea V, Di Marco C, Savino G, Tiozzo V, Catania A. Meta-analysis of randomized trials on the efficacy of vascular closure devices after diagnostic angiography and angioplasty. Am Heart J. 2010;159(4):518–531.

9. Vierhout BP, Saleem BR, Ott A, van Dijl JM, de Kempenaer TD van A, Pierie MEN, et al. A comparison of Percutaneous femoral access in Endovascular Repair versus Open femoral access (PiERO): study protocol for a randomized controlled trial. Trials. 2015;16:408.

10. Bertrand OF, Rao SV, Pancholy S, Jolly SS, Rodes-Cabau. J, Larose. E, et al. Transradial approach for coronary angiography and interventions: results of the First International Transradial Practice Survey. JACC Cardiovasc Interv. 2010;3(10):1022–1031.

11. Sandoval Y, Burke MN, Lobo AS, Lips DL, Seto AH, Chavez I, et al. Contemporary arterial access in the cardiac catheterization laboratory. JACC Cardiovasc Interv. 2017;10(22):2233–2241.

12. Rathore S, Stables RH, Pauriah M, Hakeem A, Mills JD, Palmer ND, et al. A randomized comparison of TR band and radistop hemostatic compression devices after transradial coronary intervention. Catheter Cardiovasc Interv. 2010;76(5):660–667.

INDEX

Page numbers in *italics* and **bold** refer to figures and tables respectively.

Printed in the United States
By Bookmasters